PROFESSIONAL DISCIPLINE IN NURSING

THEORY AND PRACTICE

PROFESSIONAL DISCIPLINE IN NURSING

THEORY AND PRACTICE

Reginald H. Pyne
SRN RFN FBIM

Deputy Registrar
General Nursing Council
for England and Wales

Blackwell Scientific Publications
OXFORD LONDON EDINBURGH
BOSTON MELBOURNE

© 1981 by
Blackwell Scientific Publications
Editorial offices:
Osney Mead, Oxford OX2 0EL
8 John Street, London WC1N 2ES
9 Forrest Road, Edinburgh EH1 2QH
52 Beacon Street, Boston
    Massachusetts 02108 USA
214 Berkeley Street, Carlton
    Victoria 3053 Australia

First published 1981

Set by Southline Press Ltd,
Ferring, Sussex
Printed and bound in Great Britain
by Billing & Sons Ltd,
Guildford, London, Oxford and Worcester

DISTRIBUTORS
USA
    Blackwell Mosby Book Distributors
    11830 Westline Industrial Drive
    St Louis, Missouri 63141

Canada
    Blackwell Mosby Book Distributors
    120 Melford Drive, Scarborough
    Ontario M1B 2X4

Australia
    Blackwell Scientific Book
    Distributors
    214 Berkeley Street, Carlton
    Victoria 3053

British Library
Cataloguing in Publication Data

Pyne, Reginald H.
    Professional discipline in nursing.
    1. Nurse – Discipline – Great Britain
    I. Title
    610.73'06'9   RT11   80–42387
    ISBN 0–632–00728–1

Contents

Preface

In 1980, the implementation of the Nurses, Midwives and Health Visitors Act of 1979 began by the creation of the United Kingdom Central Council for Nursing, Midwifery and Health Visiting, and of the National Boards for each of the four countries. With it commenced the massive task of preparing the vast quantity of statutory rules that must receive parliamentary approval before the functions of the existing statutory bodies, and those responsible for postbasic education, can be steadily absorbed, the whole process eventually resulting in the dissolution of those bodies.

So far as nursing is concerned, this means the creation of new arrangements for the regulation of the profession through the professional disciplinary process. This simple fact provides the reason for setting down in some detail the system as it has evolved for the statutory body with the largest number of registered and enrolled nurses in Great Britain. Throughout, I freely state my personal views about the strengths and weaknesses of the existing professional disciplinary process of the General Nursing Council for England and Wales, and of the range of decisions available in law to the committees whose members bear the onerous burden of this important work.

We would do well to remind ourselves that the form of statutory control of nursing that for many years we have taken for granted did not always exist. This book is not an exercise in nostalgia or reminiscence but a reminder of how precious our professional inheritance is, how hard it was won, and how great our responsibility is to the future. My intent in studying the past and reviewing the present is to provide applicable lessons towards improving the future.

In the first three chapters, I explore the concepts of profession and professional responsibility as related to nursing. Through a case-law history, I provide a background to the development of the nursing profession and its disciplinary process and show the ways in which that process has changed over the years.

The middle chapters are meant to be a handbook on professional disciplinary procedures within the United Kingdom. With my working experience in the General Nursing Council for England and Wales, I explain how a specialist professional social work service has been associated with the disciplinary function and describe the framework and structure of the statutory body and its procedures and options. I consider the sources of reports or complaints that require the attention of the Investigating and Disciplinary committees and show how those matters are sieved. In many respects, they approximate or are the same as those of the other statutory bodies responsible for nursing and midwifery in the United Kingdom.

In Chapter 7, I examine the origins and development of a professional social work agency now available and how it assists nurses who are involved in, or at risk of becoming involved in, the professional disciplinary process. This significant development has constructively influenced both the philosophy and practice of professional discipline.

In Chapter 8, I consider what lessons can be drawn from an observation and study of the professional disciplinary work of the statutory nursing bodies, and what indications emerge of problems that must be tackled as a matter of urgency if reasonable standards of nursing are to be available to the public. Many points may well be regarded as rather stern criticism: that some nurse manages fail to fulfil certain of their professional responsibilities with serious consequences resulting; that some employing authorities should look to their excessive demands or expectations of offending employees before absolving themselves of fault; that the quality of representation that staff organisations provide for their members is not always as good as those members have the right to expect; and that the procedures laid down in statutory rules and the range of decisions available to the General Nursing Council for England and Wales leave something to be desired. It is apparent that I spare no one *including* myself from criticism. I do this by giving my answers to a series of relevant questions, and continue through in Chapter 9 on new trends and implications. In the last chapter, by scrutinising some sections of the Nurses, Midwives and Health Visitors Act of 1979, I take a look at the possible future of the profession.

The Appendices provide a set of varied case studies which can be used by the individual or by study or seminar groups of nurses at all levels. At the end of each case is a series of options; the actual decisions and points for discussion follow the last case. Their ultimate aim is a deeper knowledge of professional responsibility and a greater determination to act responsibly.

Since 1973, I have addressed audiences of nurses in many parts of Great Britain on the professional disciplinary responsibilities of the

General Nursing Council for England and Wales, and the ways in which the exercise of those responsibilities, if observed, and if lessons are learnt from that observation, can become a means of preventing a general deterioration of professional standards and also of encouraging individual responsibility. I received many comments and letters after such talks; some told me that they returned to their work with eyes more alert to the hazards to be found there—hazards that endanger patients and the professional careers of the nursing staff. When they asked, 'Why don't you write a book on the subject of professional discipline and professional responsibility?', I often replied that perhaps one day I would.

Whether I would have got down to writing on the subject, important though I believe it to be, without a direct invitation to do so is doubtful. I am, therefore, extremely grateful to my publishers for inviting me to set down and develop the points I have made in the past from many platforms. I hope that this book serves as a catalyst to further valuable consideration of the various aspects of professional responsibility.

January 1981   *Reginald H. Pyne*

Acknowledgements

My task in writing this book has been made easier than would otherwise have been the case because of the encouragement, support and assistance of a number of people, and I acknowledge their various degrees of involvement. I am grateful to:

Maude Storey (the third Registrar of the General Nursing Council for England and Wales with whom I have had the privilege of working) for her general encouragement to take up this project, and for the many stimulating conversations we have shared out of which some material in this book has quietly grown.

John Maher, my friend and colleague, for contributing the main substance of the chapter on the Nurses Welfare Service, a development with which I am proud to be associated.

Sonja Wolfskehl, my colleague and personal assistant, for sharing and bearing so many of the burdens of my working life that have to do with the professional disciplinary role of the General Nursing Council for England and Wales.

Maureen, my nurse wife, for reading and giving her opinions of substantial parts of my text.

The editors of *Nursing Times* and *Nursing Mirror*, respectively, for permission to reproduce their leading articles of 2 August 1979.

The General Nursing Council for England and Wales, my employers, for permission to reproduce certain of their documents which have an obvious relationship to the subject of this book and for the privilege that has been mine of working as their senior officer in the sphere of professional discipline. (With the exception of the quotations from Council reports, circulars, and the like, the views expressed are *my own*.)

Most of all, I am grateful to my excellent secretary, *Diana Barden*, for converting my badly written manuscript into her usual attractively typed format with the minimum of errors and with negligible delay.

1

What is a Profession?

What is a profession? What does membership of a profession involve? What is professional responsibility? Can nursing honestly claim to be a profession? These questions are often posed by people with enquiring minds, but the answers that they receive are not always adequate. I believe that nursing can justly claim to be a profession for reasons that I trust will become clear as the pages of this book are turned.

As for the other questions, after nearly a decade of employment in a post which has required me to operate the system whereby the profession of nursing in England and Wales is to some extent regulated through the statutory body's professional disciplinary process, I have come to the firm conclusion that consideration of some negative aspects (e.g., professional misconduct; professional negligence; professional irresponsibility) often helps to provide clues to the most satisfactory answers. Let me illustrate what I mean.

CASE 1

In 1975, notification was received by the General Nursing Council for England and Wales that a state enrolled nurse, aged 21 years, had been convicted in court of theft of drugs and unlawful possession of drugs. She had pleaded guilty to the offence, and the decision of the court was to discharge her conditionally for 12 months.
She started a nursing career in 1972, following a period of dissatisfaction and restlessness in other work. That restlessness soon disappeared, and she seemed to have found her niche.
The incident that led to her appearance in court occurred shortly after a holiday on the Continent. The nurse returned from the sort of good holiday that leaves you feeling very tired, and almost in need of another but more restful holiday. She returned to her hospital work, and on only her second day back she was approached by a porter on the staff who was known to her, but only as a passing acquaintance. He said to her that she looked tired. She agreed, and said it was the result of the pleasant but extremely demanding holiday she had just

1

enjoyed. He offered her a tablet which he said would 'pick her up'; unwisely she took it. It was an amphetamine tablet.

One or two days later the same man approached her, and indicated that, as a qualified nurse, she should not have taken the drug from him and as she had he could get her into a great deal of trouble. He said he would not do so provided she obtain more drugs for him. In a state of fear and anxiety this is exactly what she did. Her offences at this time included the forgery of some prescriptions for Tenuate Dospan.

For several days this continued, and the nurse worried about it a great deal. Fortunately she lived at home, where she enjoyed a good relationship with her mother. She at last managed to tell her mother, whose reaction was, 'We're not having any of that, my girl!' She then took her to the senior nursing officer of the hospital and also to the police to bring the subject completely into the open. In consequence of this action the police were able to detain the porter, a person who in their eyes was a much more serious offender. Although they had to take the matter to the Magistrates' Court, as a result of their submissions the decision of the Court was a very lenient one. The view of the employers was not. Even though there had been nothing to suggest that the nurse's conduct and performance previously had been anything other than extremely satisfactory, she was dismissed from her employment.

The Investigating Committee of the General Nursing Council for England and Wales forwarded this case for a hearing before the Disciplinary Committee. The nurse attended with her mother. The nurse was entirely open with the Committee, and answered their questions in a way that convinced them that she was a basically sensible and extremely caring girl. She was certainly aware of the significance of the mistake she had made, and was most contrite. She indicated her anxiety to continue her career in nursing, and expressed the view that she had much to offer. To the Committee she seemed exactly the sort of person they would expect never to find in this position. By the time of the hearing she had obtained employment in a smaller geriatric hospital (from whose senior nursing officer, having knowledge of the facts, there came an excellent reference) and was clearly enjoying caring for old people very much.

The members of the Disciplinary Committee had to decide if the offence reported constituted professional misconduct and, if so, whether they could leave this nurse with the right to practise in her profession. Case 1 says a number of things that might help us to approach some answers to the original questions. For instance, it illustrates that nurses are subject to the law of the land in the same way as other members of the public. But it goes further than that by illustrating that professional nurses who offend in this way will also be subject to the judgement of their colleagues who, acting on behalf of the profession, have to consider their appropriateness to continue as members of the profession with all its privileges and responsibilities. This case also makes the point that such a consideration about a nurse's professional status is not dependent upon and need not be delayed for any decisions of the employer to retain in employment or dismiss a qualified nurse. (In case 1 the Disciplinary Committee did consider the matter 'professional misconduct', administered a severe caution, but took no other disciplinary action.)

The matters raised in case 1 may be taken a step further by consideration of another case.

CASE 2

In 1976 a report was received from a district nursing officer in respect of a state registered nurse employed as a theatre sister. Following enquiries initiated by a consultant anaesthetist the nurse admitted that she had misappropriated two 100 mg ampoules of pethidine from the theatre stock, and made fictitious entries in the drug register (including forged signatures) to cover that misappropriation.
When in possession of her admission in writing the district nursing officer dismissed her from employment and reported the matter to the police. Although her admission was not retracted the police did not bring charges because the monetary value of the drugs was so small. (It would have been less than 5 pence at the time.)
She then appealed against dismissal, and was reinstated by an appeal committee of the Area Health Authority because the police had not charged her with a criminal offence. At this stage the district nursing officer placed the nurse on suspension from duty, reported the facts to the General Nursing Council for England and Wales so that they could be considered as allegations of professional misconduct, and awaited the outcome.

Again case 2 makes the point that a decision about a person's status as an employee cannot preempt the profession's decision about that person's status as a nurse. It illustrates that nurse managers who allow that to happen by not reporting such matters abrogate their personal professional responsibility. Case 2 also indicates that the statutory body with responsibility to determine what, in a particular set of circumstances, is professional misconduct are not dependent on the criminal courts to establish guilt, but are able to consider the facts and arrive at appropriate conclusions themselves. (In case 2 the Disciplinary Committee considered the admitted facts to be professional misconduct, and removed her name from the Register of Nurses.)
Let us consider just one more case before turning again to the original series of questions.

CASE 3

In February 1979, in the High Court of Justice, the lord chief justice

and two other judges considered an appeal against a decision of the Disciplinary Committee of the General Nursing Council for England and Wales to remove a nurse from the Register of Nurses. That decision had been taken at the conclusion of a long and careful hearing in April 1978.
The man concerned held SRN and RMN qualifications. At the time of the incident he was employed in the psychiatric unit of a district general hospital. He was removed from the Register, the allegations against him having been proved to the Disciplinary Committee's satisfaction, on what must be the ultimate in professional charges of 'failing to give appropriate care to a patient in his charge'.

Case 3 is quoted not because the lord chief justice and his colleagues dismissed the appeal but because in doing so they made it quite clear that they would only consider whether a reasonable group of people, faced with the evidence that was given, could find the allegations proved beyond reasonable doubt. Further, in establishing their support for the conclusion that the allegations were proved, they saw it as no part of their role to question the decision of a professional committee, primarily composed of practising nurses, who had resolved that: the facts did constitute professional misconduct and removal from the Register of Nurses was the appropriate judgement.

So even the eminent judges of the High Court accept that the nursing profession, through its statutory framework, has to make its own decisions as to the sort of conduct that warrants removal of the right to practice from a nurse.

Now let us look again at the questions that opened this chapter. What is a profession? What does membership of a profession involve? What is professional responsibility? Can nursing honestly claim to be a profession?

Dictionaries are the obvious source of definitions, but sadly, in respect of any attempt to grasp the concept of a profession, they are not entirely adequate. The word is more often defined as relating to the vows of a religious community than to any areas of employment, just as the word *professional* seems (in the way it is defined) to have to do more with participating in sport for gain than with membership of a body of people who recognise and adhere to certain ethical standards. However, a study of the dictionaries is certainly not a wasted exercise. The following phrases have been extracted from the definitions of the word *profession*:

A calling requiring specialised knowledge and often long and intensive academic preparation [*Webster's New Collegiate Dictionary*, 1980].

A vocation in which a professed knowledge of some department of learning is used in its application to the affairs of others, or in the practice of an art founded upon it [*The Shorter Oxford English Dictionary*, 1973].

Occupation requiring training and intellectual abilities, practised so as to earn a living [*The Penguin English Dictionary*, 1965].

An employment not mechanical and requiring some degree of learning [*Chambers Twentieth Century Dictionary*, 1972].

An occupation , especially one that involves knowledge and training in a branch of advanced learning [*The Oxford Paperback Dictionary*, 1979].

If, like me, you find the above extracts woefully inadequate as you seek to apply them to the art and science of nursing I suggest you note that they seem equally inadequate when applied to other health professions. One might expect that a study of the definitions of *professionalism* would prove valuable, but it does not because it constantly relates back to what (for my present purpose) are the inadequate or unsatisfactory definitions of *profession*.

So where else can we turn for assistance as we attempt to grasp (in the fullest sense of the word) the concept of a profession, and to provide criteria against which to measure this occupation or vocation that we call nursing? There may be many other sources, but I turn only to one, because for me, though extremely succinct, it is also comprehensive. In a letter to the *Daily Telegraph* that was published on 12 September 1978, J. Ralph Blanchfield first commented on the abuse of the term *profession* and the need to define it, and then continued:

'Profession' cannot be defined in terms of any single characteristic. To justify the description, an occupational group must fulfil not some but all of the following criteria:
1. Its practice is based on a recognised body of learning.
2. It establishes an independent body for the collective pursuit of aims and objects related to these criteria.
3. Admission to corporate membership is based on strict standards of competence attested by examinations and assessed experience.
4. It recognises that its practice must be for the benefit of the public as well as that of the practitioners.
5. It recognises its responsibility to advance and extend the body of learning on which it is based.
6. It recognises its responsibility to concern itself with facilities, methods and provision for educating and training future entrants and for enhancing the knowledge of present practitioners.

7. It recognises the need for its members to conform to high
standards of ethics and professional conduct set out in a published
code with appropriate disciplinary procedures.

Does this improve on the definitions drawn from a selection of
dictionaries? Surely the answer is Yes. The dictionaries variously
described the role as calling, vocation, occupation and employment.
They also refer variously to the specialised knowledge, academic preparation, department of learning, training and knowledge on which it is
based. In this respect they compare only with the first of the seven
points in the letter quoted. Ironically it is on this very point that some
people argue that nursing is not a profession. Nursing (they say) cannot
be regarded as a profession, because it is based not on a body of
knowledge of its own but on that of the medical profession.

Whilst I readily accept that much of the nurse's role is concerned
with the administration of drugs and the provision of treatment prescribed by doctors, there is very much more to nursing than that. I feel
sure that any patients who received only the treatment prescribed by
doctors would feel very aggrieved. The many other things that go to
make nursing what it is are based on a body of knowledge and practical
skill which, while often applied as a complement to prescribed medical
treatment and drugs, can stand and often does stand on its own. On this
knowledge and these skills those who aspire to be registered or enrolled nurses are examined. It is therefore my contention that nursing
fulfills the first criterion of the Blanchfield definition.

What of the other criteria? The second is met by the existence (in
accordance with statute) of the General Nursing Council for England
and Wales, the General Nursing Council for Scotland, and the Northern Ireland Council for Nurses and Midwives, all soon to be phased out
as the new bodies to be established under the terms of the Nurses,
Midwives and Health Visitors Act take on their present functions, and
those of certain other existing statutory and non-statutory bodies. The
third criterion is fulfilled by the nursing councils being as satisfied as is
possible, in accordance with the statutes, with the competence of those
they admit to the Register or Roll of Nurses in the countries that make
up the United Kingdom.

The basis of the response to the fourth criterion has been enshrined
in law since the Nurses Registration Act of 1919, and it is but a
statement of fact to record that the majority of the qualified practitioners of nursing readily accept the truth of this statement. The fifth and
sixth criteria, while always receiving some attention, have (perhaps)
received less attention in the past than was deserved. Happily this has
been changing for the better in recent years as more evidence of valid

nursing research has been seen, as the increased membership of nursing and health service staff organisations had led to more articulate and comprehensive expression of concern at any shortfall in both these respects, and as individual nurses have become more aware of the fact that their personal professional responsibility extends into these areas.

As for the last of the seven criteria, nursing most certainly qualifies. This is illustrated by the remaining chapters of this book. The over-all aim is twofold: to disseminate information on the ways in which the nursing profession regulates itself and to stimulate discussion which will foster individual and collective professional development.

Having agreed that nursing is a profession according to the seven-point definition the reader might assume that I accept it as a perfect definition, but that is not the case. There are a number of respects in which I would dispute the wording to some small degree, but it would be a difference of a semantic nature rather than of principle. However, I would have preferred to see the fourth point more strongly worded. For me, one of the hallmarks of a profession is that it exists as a result of legislation that is designed for the protection of the public, but for operation by the profession itself. This is most certainly the case with nursing in the United Kingdom, and it is something precious which the members of the profession must safeguard.

So much for the first (What is a profession?) and fourth (Can nursing honestly claim to be a profession?) opening questions. What of the other two? On reflection I think that these are two facets of the same point. From time to time I am invited to speak to meetings of nurse managers on the subject of 'The responsibility of the nurse manager'. I think that on occasions I disappoint those who have been responsible for the invitation by expounding the view that, with one or two aspects rather more intensely developed, the professional responsibilities of the nurse manager are those that accrue to any qualified nurse, no matter what post he or she may be filling. These professional responsibilities I believe, in essence to be:

a. Any registered or enrolled nurse has a responsibility for his or her own standards of nursing care, and for his or her skills, attitudes and qualities of observation.

b. Any registered or enrolled nurse has a responsibility to participate in the teaching of others.

c. Any registered or enrolled nurse has a measure of responsibility for the setting in which patients are cared for.

d. Any registered or enrolled nurse has a responsibility to care for and about his or her colleagues.

I readily accept that the responsibilities referred to in points *b* and *c* become greater for those who take up certain specialised teaching or managerial posts, but this should not be allowed to absolve all other qualified nurses from their responsibility, just as the existence of occupational health departments and personnel nurses should not absolve them from their personal responsibilities under *d*. It would be churlish of me to imply or suggest that the responsibilities of the nurse managers go no further than that, though I would argue that the various ways in which their responsibilities are greater are basically extensions of the points made as *a* to *d*.

So what are the additional professional responsibilities of the nurse as a manager? I suggest four points, which are presented as complementing each other, rather than as having an order of importance:

1. Nurse managers have a responsibility to create, maintain and sustain a setting which is dynamic, so that nurses (not only those in training) may grow and improve, and thus contribute to the growth and improvement of others.

This is not only (indeed not even mainly) about equipment but much more about attitudes.

2. Nurse managers have a responsibility to the public to ensure that those they employ as qualified nurses *are* qualified nurses.

The simple presentation of a certificate proves nothing, since many hundreds of nurses each year report the loss of their certificates and seek replacements. Nurse managers should invariably check with the appropriate Council about the continuing validity of those certificates, and invariably do all other things that they can to ensure that the presenter of a valid certificate is its owner before taking that person into employment. As an employer of nurses it is dangerous to assume anything!

3. Nurse managers have a responsibility for the settings in which patients are nursed.

I appreciate that this echoes point *c*, but I repeat it without apology for the nurse managers' responsibility is greater. It is a responsibility that they must bear not only that patients may receive the safe and competent nursing care they deserve but that nurses working in those settings are not rendered vulnerable by excessive and unreasonable pressure.

4. Nurse managers have a responsibility to recognise that they have certain personal professional responsibilities that they cannot and must not abrogate to others.

These, then, are in my view the responsibilities that accrue first to all qualified nurses and second to those who take on the burdens of management. You may not necessarily agree with my lists. If you do not I respect your right to come to different conclusions in producing your own answers to the question What is professional responsibility? If my conclusions do not appeal to you I suggest that, without delay, you prepare a list for yourself. I hope and believe that, as it does with me, it will lead you to the conclusion that the nursing profession, through each and every one of its members, must come to recognise its collective responsibility for regulating itself. While a special and substantial part of that responsibility is laid by the law of the land on the relevant statutory bodies (through their power in respect of individuals and institutions), the remaining part, and undoubtedly the largest part, must come from the self-discipline of the profession's members. Without that, no matter how we may define the word *profession*, we shall not deserve that honoured title. (Appendix A contains further case studies which relate to the subject matter of this chapter.)

REFERENCES

Webster's New Collegiate Dictionary, Eighth Edition (1980). Springfield, Mass.: G. & C. Merriam Co. By permission. From *Webster's New Collegiate Dictionary* © 1980 by G. & C. Merriam Co., Publishers of the Merriam-Webster Dictionaries.

The Shorter Oxford English Dictionary, Third Edition (1973). Edited by C. T. Onions. Oxford: Oxford University Press. Excerpt reprinted by permission of Oxford University Press.

The Penguin English Dictionary (1969). Edited by G. N. Garmonsay & J. Simpson. Harmondsworth: Penguin Books. Reprinted by permission of Penguin Books.

Chambers Twentieth Century Dictionary (1972). Edited by A. M. Macdonald. Edinburgh & London: W. & R. Chambers Ltd.

The Oxford Paperback Dictionary (1979). Edited by J. M. Hawkins. Oxford: Oxford University Press. Excerpt reprinted by permission of Oxford University Press.

2

The Concept of Professional Discipline

What is professional discipline? Is it concerned with professional ethics or conduct or standards of practice?

Possibly these questions, as with the questions asked at the beginning of Chapter 1, may be best approached by considering first a negative aspect of the subject. I do not mean that we should, at this stage, consider the consequences of a lack of discipline on the part of members of the nursing profession; the concerns I have about that lack and the evidence on which those concerns are based will emerge gradually. The negative aspect that I have in mind is rather that as we educate nurses in those theoretical and practical aspects contained in the scheme of training and as we introduce them to the role that they must fulfil as qualified nurses, we so often fail to develop in them an understanding of what professional responsibility means. Let me try to illustrate part of what I mean:

CASE 4

> In 1978 a registered mental nurse appeared before the Disciplinary Committee of the General Nursing Council for England and Wales following a conviction in a criminal court for cultivating cannabis plants at his home, and for having various drugs in his possession that were the property of the hospital at which he had been employed. (These items were expectorants, mild analgesics, and vitamins.)
> At a certain stage of the hearing a Committee member asked him how he viewed the matter in retrospect, and (like so many others in similar positions over the years) he gave an answer which was based only on the effect that it had had on his life, with no apparent thought for or understanding of the significance of his contravention of the law or his self-medication. 'Well' he said, 'I was foolish really. I had a good job, quite near to home, and not bad pay, and now I've lost it all'.

Consider the way in which case 5 illustrates the same failure to understand what professional responsibility means:

10

CASE 5

The General Nursing Council for England and Wales were notified by the police that a registered nurse (SRN, RMN) had appeared in a Magistrates' Court and pleaded guilty to a charge of criminal deception, having on two occasions dishonestly obtained a quantity of Brufen tablets from the hospital in which he had been employed as a charge nurse. The magistrates imposed a conditional discharge for one year, and his employers dismissed him from his post.

Now the relevant committees of the Council had to make their judgement on him as a registered nurse, bearing in mind the nature of the offence to which he had pleaded guilty, and (of course) such evidence as they had available to them about his career to that date, supplemented finally by the impressions they were able to form out of their own personal experience.

The circumstances (as put to the Disciplinary Committee on behalf of the nurse) had been that the nurse had a close friend who suffered from rheumatoid arthritis, for which Brufen had previously been prescribed. The friend had consumed all the prescribed tablets and, having taken considerable time off from his work due to his condition and wishing to avoid further absence that would be necessary were he to visit his doctor (the Committee were told), asked his friend the charge nurse if he could obtain a supply of the drug for him. It appeared that the nurse readily agreed to the request, and the friend agreed to collect the tablets from him at the hospital two days later. To obtain the supply the nurse made out a patient's treatment chart for a non-existent patient and signed it himself, copying a doctor's signature. He then sent it to the pharmacy with the normal ward orders, ensuring he would be available when the supply was returned to the ward and would empty the box. Having obtained this first supply the nurse said he put them into his pocket to keep them on his person for safety. Unfortunately (for him), on the day when his friend called to collect the tablets he had (it was said on his behalf) left them at home. Not wanting to let his friend down, he quickly repeated the procedure, obtained more tablets, and gave them to his friend.

It became apparent in the course of the hearing that the matter came to light because the nurse then left the second 'fictitious' patient's treatment chart on his desk where it was seen by the doctor whose signature had been copied, whereupon he contacted the senior nursing officer. One other disturbing point to emerge in the course of the hearing was that the nurse appeared to know very little of the nature of the drug he had fraudulently obtained.

[The reader might care to consider which of the available decisions he or she would consider appropriate in cases 4 and 5 after learning of the options available to the Disciplinary Committee. Those options are presented and explained in Chapter 6.]

Were the nurses who were the subjects of cases 4 and 5 guilty (in professional terms) of indiscipline or irresponsibility? Are these the same thing? Perhaps we should turn to the same dictionaries again to assist in arriving at some definition of our terms; first *Discipline*. Unfortunately, they provide me with no more assistance in respect of this word than they did with the word *profession*, discussed in chapter 1. I say this because (where the word is used as a noun) it tends for the most part to be indentified with other words or phrases that do not really approach the interpretation that members of recognised professions would seek. For example, the word is identified as 'instruction', 'order', 'mortification', 'punishment', 'training that moulds the mental faculties', 'training in the practice of arms', etc. While I am sure that all these words and phrases are valid in defining *discipline*, they do not satisfy my requirements as I search for an explanation of 'professional discipline'.

Buried within the larger definitions, however, there are again some points that do help, even if they are not entirely satisfactory; for instance, 'mode of life in accordance with rules'; 'orderly or prescribed pattern of behaviour'; 'a rule or system of rules governing conduct or activity'; 'a system of rules for conduct'; and 'self control'.

All of that does, I believe, take us forward at least a little. If I have to particularise why I am not entirely satisfied I would have to say that it is because of the emphasis on *rules*. In respect of any occupational or vocational group which can rightly claim the name 'profession' I maintain that rules are concerned with the structure within which the profession is managed and operates, and should not be used to define acceptable or unacceptable behaviour. What is acceptable or unacceptable behaviour has to be decided by considering it in its context.

Over the years I have become convinced that to respond to the pressures that are often applied to define professional misconduct in nursing by producing a list of proscribed actions would be dangerous, since the circumstances in which incidents that raise the question Is this professional misconduct? are rarely the same. To enshrine in statutory rules a list of actions (or inactions) that are considered professional misconduct would be bad both for members of the profession and for the public.

It would be unsatisfactory for the members of the profession as the context of an alleged offence (often unreasonable by virtue of excessive pressure of work, unclear policies, inadequate management, etc.) would not be able to be taken into account before labelling a piece of behaviour 'professional misconduct'. For the public who depend on the availability of a competent and caring nursing service it would be unsatisfactory because no list prepared now could cater for all possible eventualities in 10 years' time. If such a list had been prepared in 1970 who could have imagined that by 1980 it would be sadly lacking for its omission of any reference to putting patients at risk by any sudden withdrawal of service? The inevitable conclusion drawn by those faced with the task of producing such a list would be that it had to be couched in such general terms that it would be better to have no such document at all. Besides, would such a closely defined set of rules on 'misconduct' (even if it could be kept up to date, which is unlikely in the extreme) be consistent with membership of a profession whose practitioners must be constantly engaged in the exercise of personal judgement and responsibility, and in an often imperfect environment?

Now, let us direct our attention to the second word, *responsibility*, because I have used it frequently and shall continue to do so. Here I find my dictionaries much more to my liking, since they clearly indicate (a) that to be responsible is to be obliged either legally or morally to take care of something or to carry out a duty and (b) that one is liable to be blamed for failure. Surely these are things about which professional nurses know a great deal and which, as part of their professional calling, they readily accept.

Lack of responsibility, however, is not something that is manifested only by nurses who work in clinical settings. Those who have accepted the additional responsibilities of working as nurse managers often reveal it just as strongly. When that happens the consequences may be still more serious, because the nurse manager who fails to act responsibly not only affects for ill the service to patients but creates a situation in which his or her own staff may be put at risk. And the consequences may be made heavier still if a decision is made which seeks a short-term solution to a problem with no thought for the long-term consequences. Let me illustrate in case 6 what I mean.

CASE 6

The Investigating Committee of the General Nursing Council for England and Wales had to consider documentary evidence put before them in respect of a 33-year-old SRN employed as sister-in-charge of an intensive care unit who had been found staggering about on the unit early one afternoon, and admitted that she had ingested two or three sodium amytal tablets which had been taken from a partly empty bottle that had been in the possession of a patient admitted earlier that day.

On the face of it this appeared to be a serious failure on the part of the nurse concerned. However, the background picture showed that the greater failure was that of her managers.

It emerged that (some months before) the nursing officer to whom this SRN had a line responsibility had to be admitted to hospital for a planned major operation, and it was known that she would be absent from her duties for some months. There being no spare staff available for cover, the nurse managers took stock of their position and, having agreed that this SRN was very reliable, decided that they would concentrate their resources on covering the absent nursing officer's duties in those areas where the ward sisters were less reliable or experienced.

With her link to more senior management gone (because of the absence of the nursing officer in whom she had great confidence and with whom she had a good working relationship), the sister found that the pressure on her increased as the intensive care unit became progressively more busy, there was severe staff shortage and little continuity, and the staff she did have were often of inadequate quality or experience. Being the sort of person she was, this nurse began to work quite excessive hours to keep the unit going, and even stopped leaving the unit for meal breaks. Nobody seemed to notice the stresses to which she was being subjected, or how excessively tired she appeared.

On the day of the incident the nurse once again did not leave the unit for lunch but simply snatched a few minutes for a cup of coffee in the staff room. It was at this time that she ingested the tablets which (inevitably in view of her tired condition) had a speedy effect. She tried to return to her duties, but was seen staggering about by another nurse who called the senior nursing officer for assistance. Then the more senior nurse managers became aware of just how great were the burdens that this nurse had borne (so great indeed that when they had to manage without her they found it necessary to close the unit).

With the full picture seen and understood the managers were both kind and helpful, in that they channelled her to appropriate medical help, and reassured her about her future employment with them when she was well again. While the appropriate nurse manager reported the matter to the Council so that the nurse's actions could be subject to consideration about her future as a registered nurse, she readily accepted that they had failed the nurse, and asked for the early support of one of the professional social workers of the Nurses Welfare Service. [This service is described in Chapter 7.]

At least in case 6 the managers recognised that they also had failed, and undoubtedly learnt from the unfortunate experience. It is not always so as case 7 may illustrate.

CASE 7

A 28-year-old SRN was reported to the General Nursing Council for England and Wales by the police following a conviction in a Magistrates' Court for stealing considerable quantities of pethidine and Fortral, together with syringes and needles, from the company for which she worked as an industrial nurse.

The nurse was able to meet a professional social worker from the Nurses Welfare Service in advance of the Disciplinary Committee hearing, and as a result she clearly understood the role of that

Committee, and appreciated that a decision to remove her from the Register of Nurses (if it were made) would serve to protect the public and would be a positive contribution to her rehabilitation, since she would find it difficult to break her dependence on drugs so easily accessible to a qualified nurse. The Disciplinary Committee did resolve to remove her name from the Register, but she left the room not feeling punished, as eventual restoration was the target towards which she could aim with continuing support and guidance of a professional social worker with detailed knowledge of her problem. However, the still more significant and disturbing feature of case 7 lies in the fact that it could have so easily been avoided if only a group of nurse managers had taken appropriate action a year earlier.

One of the documents assembled for the consideration of this case was a copy of the psychiatrist's report prepared for the Magistrates' Court. One crucial phrase which leapt from the pages of that report was to the effect that one year earlier, when employed as a ward sister, she had been discovered misappropriating diazepam from her ward stock, and had been quietly asked to resign, in return for which they (the nurse managers) would take no further action on the matter. She did resign, and very quickly found new employment in a heavy engineering company, where controlled drugs were (of necessity) available, and where the control system was grossly inadequate. The consequences you now know.

Case 7 is one which the nurse concerned was not the only one who failed to act responsibly. The nurse managers also have much to answer for, since, in seeking a short-term solution to their immediate problem (at the time of the diazepam incident), and thus avoiding any bad publicity for 'their hospital', they abrogated most aspects of their professional responsibility. In disposing of this particular nurse from their employment but not reporting her to the Council, they were simply (to put the best possible interpretation on it) acting to protect their particular patients at that time. In so doing, however, they were neglecting their responsibilities to patients and the public as a whole; they were neglecting their responsibilities to the nursing profession and its standards; and they were neglecting their responsibilities to this sick member of their profession. By their failure the public were put at risk, and this sick colleague was allowed to become more drug dependent, requiring more time and much more medical and social work assistance for her rehabilitation.

While professional nurses undoubtedly are responsible for their own actions and nurse managers have additional responsibilities which relate to both the public and the members of the profession (and which must be exercised with both short-term and long-term consequences in mind), all members of the profession have a responsibility for each other.

Unfortunately all too often it seems that we choose to look the other way or to 'not interfere' when we suspect that a colleague is behaving unprofessionally. Quite apart from possibly putting himself or herself in professional jeopardy, the nurse constitutes a risk to patients if he or she becomes an unsafe practitioner. Qualified nurses, by their unquestioning response to certain requests and by their willingess to disregard carefully prepared policies, so often unwittingly fail their patients, their profession, and their colleagues. Just one more illustration must suffice.

CASE 8

A staff nurse on night duty expressed concern at the fact that another registered nurse was borrowing pethidine from her ward very often, and suggested that the stock on that ward must be inadequate. This innocent report led to an investigation which revealed that another registered nurse had not only been obtaining pethidine from that ward, but from many other wards in this large hospital. Still more, it revealed that the 'borrowing' was taking place when the stock on the nurse's ward was adequate, that the patients named in the drug records did not exist, and that fictitious treatment cards had been presented. This very large quantity of pethidine (over a period of months) was illegally and fraudulently obtained by the simple expedient of going to other wards with treatment cards of non-existent patients, and stating 'I have to give this patient some pethidine, and I have run out. Can I borrow some?'
In ward after ward other qualified nurses were providing the pethidine, recording the entry in their ward controlled drugs register, signing as having witnessed the administration of the drug although they had no intention of doing so, and allowing the nurse to go from their wards with an ampoule of pethidine. In some instances the procedure was repeated with the same ward three times in the course of a single night, and all this in spite of a specific and freely available policy document on drug administration which made it clear that no controlled drug should be recorded as having been administered until it had been and that the signing of the 'witnessed' column should indicate that the administration of the drug had been witnessed and not just removed from the drug cupboard.
So much for personal responsibility for one's actions!

So what is professional discipline? Surely it is two things. At the individual level I believe it to be the self-discipline of the members of the nursing profession—their individual determination to act with responsibility and in accordance with the moral principles of their profession. At the collective level I believe it to be the process by which the nursing profession (acting on behalf of the public) operate that section of the law that permits the application of appropriate sanctions to its culpable members.

Professional discipline is also inextricably entwined with the whole theme of responsibility. I have written these words within a few days of reading an article in the *Nursing Mirror* (10/1/80), in which Baroness McFarlane of Llandaff, Professor of Nursing at the University of Manchester, wrote of her hopes for the nursing profession in the new decade. As is invariably the case, her words informed, stimulated and challenged me. She built the article around eight words; one I have already used a great deal—*responsibility*. Baroness McFarlane maintains that

> We also have a responsibility for our own professional actions. This is
> legally a fact, but as professionals we make decisions about the
> nursing care of individuals and we must be seen to be accountable for
> the clinical decisions we make and the actions we carry out. A
> developing sense of professional responsibility and accountability for
> clinical nursing actions by the practising nurse are priorities as we
> enter the next decade.

I was delighted to read such a positive statement, since we so often think and speak in negative terms when the subject is 'discipline'. or indeed 'responsibility'. To be self-disciplined and to act responsibly are positive virtues, and without them all the knowledge and skill we may possess will consistently fail to provide nursing care of a high standard. (Appendix A contains further case studies which relate to the subject matter of this chapter.)

3

The Origins of Nurse Registration
and the Regulation of
the Nursing Profession

The registration of nurses in the United Kingdom dates from 1919, when the Nurses Registration Act received the Royal Assent, and the nursing councils were established. This was the culmination of a battle of 45 years' duration. The fascinating details of those years and of the traumatic first few years of the life of the General Nursing Council for England and Wales are described in the books listed at the end of the chapter, to which the enthusiastic student of legislation can refer. It is not my purpose to duplicate that work. Nonetheless, it is worth recording that many of the items that featured in that original Act also feature in the present Nurses Acts, and in the Nurses, Midwives and Health Visitors Act of 1979; one of them is professional discipline.

Thus, from the beginning of a new regime for training, examinations, and approval of training institutions, a council with a majority of nurses also took responsibility in law for acting in the public interest by operating the procedures of professional discipline. Peer judgement had arrived, and it would be primarily nurses who would make judgements that would remove from a colleague his or her right to practise as a registered nurse. (Similar arrangements for the enrolled nurse date from the 1943 Act.) From that time onwards the Council exercised this important function on behalf of both profession and public.

At first, and indeed for many years in the case of England and Wales, the General Nursing Council considered those cases referred for a disciplinary hearing at its full Council meeting, all cases having first been considered by the Disciplinary and Penal Cases Committee who had to decide whether (in the view of the members) a prima facie case of misconduct had been established. (From the introduction of the state enrolled assistant nurse, later the state enrolled nurse, by the 1943 Nurses Act, until such nurses were accorded a full Council membership status by the 1969 Nurses Act, enrolled nurse cases were heard by the Enrolled Nurses Committee.) The disadvantage of this

18

system is clear in retrospect. When a case was forwarded for a hearing, those members already aware of the circumstances because of their membership on the Disciplinary and Penal Cases Committee would now participate in judgement of that same case—an aspect seen to be unsatisfactory over the years. Eventually, the 1969 Act ensured (for both registered and enrolled nurses) that if a case were to go right through the professional disciplinary system it would be subjected to the consideration of two entirely separate groups of members.

The records of the Disciplinary and Penal Cases Committee over the early years of the life of the General Nursing Council for England and Wales make very interesting reading, as do the Council minutes which record the charges against nurses whose cases had been forwarded for hearings by the Committee and the decisions that resulted from those hearings. They present a fragment of rather specialised social history, and reveal something of the attitudes of the members of this new profession to their delinquent peers.

What type of reports were the Disciplinary and Penal Cases Committee receiving and considering in the 1920s and 1930s? Which of them were going on to Council for hearings that would determine whether the nurses concerned might retain the right to the title of registered nurse? And, what of the decisions that Council were making about those individual nurses whose cases were forwarded to them for a hearing—Were they harsh or lenient? Were they necessary to protect the public or rather to pronounce a moral judgement or even to punish? From the records of the first thirty cases considered by the Disciplinary and Penal Cases Committee (most of which were referred to Council for subsequent consideration), we may draw our answers.

Theft from shops

We so often seem to assume that 'shoplifting' is a phenomenon of post-Second World War society; one that has to do with the emergence of tempting displays in large department stores and food supermarkets, and which dates from the time when there was no longer a counter between the customer and the goods. Twelve of the first thirty cases reported to the General Nursing Council for England and Wales following the introduction of registration of nurses (during a period commencing 1925), however, involved theft from shops. Presumably the sale arrangements for food were safer, since all these cases involved convictions for the theft of clothing; five were ladies' hats from the same large London store, and the remainder were hats (again), gloves, stockings and underclothes.

All these cases were sent to the Council, and with the exception of one (where the respondent nurse was placed on postponed judgement) the nurses were removed from the Register. It is interesting to note that the only nurse not removed was a deputy to a matron; from the matron, the chairman of the board (a magistrate who also came to the hearing), and senior medical staff, powerful written submissions in mitigation were received. Such evidence of rallying round in support of a convicted nurse, rather than dismissing her instantly, would seem to have been rare in the early days of nurse registration and the consequential professional discipline.

Questions arising from personal conduct

The reader who refers to Appendix C for a measure of comparison will not locate many offences that could be placed under this heading. Seven of the first thirty cases reported and considered, however, fall within questions arising from personal conduct.

CHARGE	DECISION
Betting in a public house	Warned about behaviour
Desertion of his wife	No action taken
Bore two illegitimate children	Removed from the Register
Living in adultery	Removed from the Register
Misconduct with a man in a hotel	Removed from the Register
Convicted of making an unauthorised street collection for a good cause	Warned about behaviour. (This lady could be regarded as singularly unfortunate, in that she rattled her collecting box at the chairman of the local Watch Committee, who then prosecuted her!)
Drunk and disorderly in a public place	Removed from the Register

Offences concerning patients or their property

Of three cases, only one (the first disciplinary case handled by the

Council) involved the theft of a diamond ring and £5 from a patient in 1925, while the others involved theft of money or jewellery from the property of deceased patients. Removal from the Register resulted in all these cases.

Theft from employing authorities or colleagues

In the first thirty cases there was only one that concerned theft from a nurse's employers (it concerned food that she said was left over and was otherwise going to waste), and two that resulted from thefts from colleagues (in one case a dress, and the other a watch). All three nurses were removed from the Register.

Offences associated with obtaining employment or occurring within it

The registered nurse who was the subject of only the second disciplinary case was reported to the Council for providing a forged character reference when she was applying for a nursing post. She was removed from the Register. The other two cases involved a nurse who was drunk on duty and one asleep on duty on two consecutive nights. In both instances removal from the Register resulted.

Other thefts (not related to work)

Only one case falls under thefts not from shops or related to work. It involved a conviction for the theft of £11 from some family friends and led to removal from the Register.

Offences involving drugs

It was not until the thirtieth case and April 1931 that the Council had to deal with a case involving drugs. The particular offence is described in the Council's records as 'Taking and unlawfully possessing Morphine'. The nurse was removed from the Register.

Many conclusions can be drawn from those first thirty cases. The first point, I suggest, is the obvious one: the Removal from the Register rate was high (twenty-six of the first thirty cases). Second, many of those removed from the Register were removed for reasons which had little or nothing to do with their work.

On the latter point, I noted with great interest the external pressure to which Council were subjected as early as the third reported case.

This was the first of the cases wherein the registered nurse concerned had been convicted of stealing a hat from a London shop. The matter was reported in the press (the first time they could have said 'state registered nurse steals from London department store') and came to the notice of the Council as well as by a report from the police. Before the Disciplinary and Penal Cases Committee could consider the matter a letter was received from the secretary of one of the nurses organisations of the day, telling the Council that they *must* remove this lady from the Register. They were even told why they must remove her from the Register. The reason was *not* to protect the patients but 'to maintain the purity of the profession'. The nurse was removed but whether for the latter reason I know not. However, I note that the phrase 'to maintain the purity of the profession' slipped into the Council's language and was often used over the next few years in professional disciplinary cases.

Another significant point to note is that a very small number of the cases (in that first period of 6 years) were the result of incidents in the nurse's working situation. What conclusions might be drawn from that? Conjecture on this point is more appropriately placed in my examination of the present and the future.

Let us leap forward in time and consider a period after the end of the Second World War. A quick look again at the questions that preceded my examination of that earlier period might be helpful. Were the decisions harsh or lenient? Were the decisions those that were necessary to protect the public? to pronounce a moral judgement? or perhaps even to punish? And now that I am referring to a period that was 15 years and a World War (with all its social change) away from the previous period reviewed, we may even question 'How adequately was the context of an offence taken into consideration in making a judgement?

Sadly we cannot possibly know the answer to the last question, but I suspect from some decisions that surprised me (by their apparent leniency) that where the offence took place in a hospital the circumstances could sometimes have a mitigatory effect. As for the previous question, I suspect that some other decisions were of a punitive nature and were based on harsh moral judgements rather than on decisions as to what was necessary to protect the public, and I imagine that those Council members who made those decisions held opinions which were not unlike those of society at large. Let me illustrate my point by reference to some of the disciplinary cases that were the subject of hearings before the Council during the latter part of and shortly after the Second World War.

EXAMPLE 1

CHARGE. Stole a quantity of drugs valued at 7 shillings from the hospital where she was employed

DECISION. Postponed judgement

COMMENT. This is a category of offence much in evidence today, and nurses are often placed on Postponed Judgement or Removed. We have no knowledge of the drugs involved, but I suspect that they were probably not narcotics.

EXAMPLE 2

CHARGE. Stole twenty clothing coupons (clothes were rationed during and for some time after the war) from an office in the hospital where she was employed

DECISION. Postponed judgement

COMMENT. Fortunately, this cannot occur today, but it is easy to accept that at the time of clothes rationing it was a serious offence, and a great temptation.

EXAMPLE 3

CHARGE. Convicted of unlawfully and wilfully ill-treating a child in a manner likely to cause him unnecessary suffering

DECISION. Removed from Register of Nurses

COMMENT. The present Disciplinary Committee have made a similar decision in a case of wilful child neglect in 1979.

EXAMPLE 4

CHARGE. Guilty of four counts of criminal abortion, three similar offences taken into consideration, for which she was sentenced to 3 years penal servitude

DECISION. Removed from Register of Nurses

COMMENT. This concerns a category of offence which disappeared from the scene when the Abortion Act of 1967 took effect. There have been no such cases referred to the General Nursing Council for England and Wales since 1973.

EXAMPLE 5

CHARGE. Unlawfully procuring three grains of morphia and unlawfully supplying such morphia to another who was not authorised to be in possession of the said drug

DECISION. Cautioned

COMMENT. This seems a very surprising decision, and there must have been some powerful evidence in mitigation for it to be made.

EXAMPLE 6

CHARGE. Intoxicated on duty on several occasions

DECISION. Removed from Register of Nurses

COMMENT. This raises a subject which is of increasing concern to the Council at the present time. The decisions now are often the same.

EXAMPLE 7

CHARGE. Misconduct in that she disregarded the hospital's rules relating to nurses by, on many occasions, going out at night with male patients without permission

DECISION. Removed from Register of Nurses
COMMENT. This must remain a mystery.

EXAMPLE 8
CHARGE. Being unmarried, she gave birth to a child
DECISION. Removed from Register of Nurses
COMMENT. This would not now be referred to the Council, and if it was it would be rejected without hesitation.

EXAMPLE 9
CHARGE. Guilty at Central Criminal Court of the infanticide of her newly born child
DECISION. Removed from Register of Nurses
COMMENT. If this were to be referred, the Investigating Committee would wish to consider all available evidence about the mental health of the nurse at the time and if it were to prove a direct consequence of postnatal depression they would probably take no action.

EXAMPLE 10
CHARGE. Found guilty of stealing goods from shops
DECISION. Removed from Register of Nurses
COMMENT. The Investigating Committee now deal with a large quantity of shoplifters each year, and provided they do not persist in committing such offences dispose of the matter by admonitory letters, and by seeking reassurances about the future. Very few re-offend.

EXAMPLE 11
CHARGE. Misconduct in that a coroner's inquest had determined that the death of two infants was caused by doses of Chlorodyne administered by the nurse to quieten them, but without criminal intent
DECISION. Not proved to the satisfaction of Council, and therefore charge dismissed
COMMENT. The facts are not sufficiently known to make a comparative comment.

EXAMPLE 12
CHARGE. Convicted of conspiracy to defraud, procuring payments on forged documents, falsifying accounts, and obtaining goods by false pretences, 207 other offences being taken into consideration
DECISION. Removed from Register of Nurses
COMMENT. This seems to be an example of a deliberately dishonest person in whose hands patients and their property may not be safe. Similar examples occur today and are dealt with similarly.

EXAMPLE 13
CHARGE. Stole a quantity of hospital property valued at £4
DECISION. Removed from Register of Nurses
COMMENT. Theft of hospital property is the subject of a disturbingly large number of reports at the present time, even though many people (including even a judge or two) or organisations regard it as a perk of the job. I was about to write that while the Investigating Committee now send many such cases to the Disciplinary Committee it is unlikely that they would do so for goods to the value of £4, but

then I remembered what £4 would buy in 1946, always assuming the goods were available to buy!

EXAMPLE 14

CHARGE. Stole £5 from a patient in a private ward
DECISION. Removed from Register of Nurses
COMMENT. This is likely to produce a similar decision now.

EXAMPLE 15

CHARGE. Misconduct, in that over 4 years she had administered to herself unprescribed drugs
DECISION. Removed from Register of Nurses
COMMENT. This is likely to produce a similar decision now.

EXAMPLE 16

CHARGE. Malingering and causing self-inflicted wounds while in the course of her duties as a nurse
DECISION. Postponed judgement
COMMENT. Comparative comment is impossible without more information.

The sixteen cases set out consititute a fairly typical example of those being forwarded to the Council for disciplinary hearings in the mid-1940s. The results summarise as:

Removed	11
Postponed judgement	3
Caution	1
Not proved	1

The Removed as a percentage of the whole looks surprisingly large by comparison with the figures of recent years (see Appendix C for 1978–79 statistics), but then as now it would doubtless have been largely dependent on the facts of the case.

The selection of cases provides the opportunity to make some comparative comments based on individual issues. The reader may draw his or her own further conclusions by comparing that information with the 1978–79 statistics in Appendix C. Some general indication, however, is needed of those areas where the pattern of reports and decisions has significantly changed, and those where it has remained constant. (Comment on new areas of importance and concern are made in Chapter 9.)

One of the 1920s categories was *Theft from Shops*. This remained conspicuous in the late 1940s, and example 10 indicates that, even for a first offence, a decision to remove a nurse from the Register (or the Roll) of Nurses was often made. Many such convictions were reported in the 1970s (ninety-seven in 1978–79 alone). Appendix C, however, shows that such cases are not now forwarded for a hearing unless the nurse persistently offends. In my time as an employee of the General Nursing Council for England and Wales I have received notification of over a thousand nurses who have been convicted of first offence shoplifting, but I have yet to know of one who has moved on to either theft from patients or from their place of nursing employment. The change in the Council's attitude which the statistics reveal is based on this simple fact.

My second category from the early years of nurse registration was *Questions Arising from Personal Conduct*. Example 8 indicates that removal from the Register for bearing an illegitimate child was still occurring in the late 1940s; 'maintaining the purity of the profession' was still a force to be reckoned with. With only one exception, this category of offence has disappeared from the statistics (see Appendix C). The exception is the Drunk and Disorderly offence. I refer in Chapter 5 to the types of conviction that the police are required to report; excessive alcohol abuse is one of them. Such cases are not considered by way of exercising a moral judgement, but simply because the view is taken that if a nurse is regularly the subject of such convictions he or she may have an alcohol problem with which he or she has not come to terms, and may thereby not (for the time being) be a safe practitioner. The profession should, through the nurse members of Council, ask themselves the appropriate questions, because to do so often introduces the nurse to an additional source of help in the form of the Nurses Welfare Service (see Chapter 7).

The *Offences Concerning Patients or Their Property* persisted in the 1940s and, sad to say, does so to the present time. However, while the two periods reviewed contained examples of theft from either patients or the property of deceased patients, the more recent statistics contain much evidence of other offences involving patients. (This is explained and considered in Chapter 9.)

Next amongst my original categories of offence was *Theft from Employing Authorities or Colleagues*. There were one and two such cases respectively in the first thirty cited, and I have given examples of such offences occurring in the postwar phase. This is another category which extends into the present.

The fifth category in my original set was headed *Offences Associated with Obtaining Employment or Occurring Within It*. Reference to the statistics in Appendix C indicates that the number of these offences is larger (much larger as a percentage of the total) today than it was in the past. I believe it is because we are now more successful at pulling into the open some of those things that in the past often stayed concealed.

The various manifestations of *Other Acts of Theft* (i.e., not concerned with patients or places of employment) or obtaining money by deception continue to appear, possibly more now than in the past because of the abundance of cheque books, credit cards, and other credit facilities in circulation.

The final category from the early years of the Council's existence was *Offences Involving Drugs*. It provided only one case in the first thirty, but the picture changed in the postwar years, and has continued to change so that over 35 per cent of the offences considered by the Disciplinary Committee of the General Nursing Council for England and Wales in 1978–79 involved drugs.

The general conclusion that I draw is that cases involving personal morality either are no longer reported or are largely disregarded, whereas the Council does increasingly hear about and get involved in matters clearly related to the delivery of safe and competent nursing care. This aspect is explored in more detail later.

In light of all that has preceded, we might consider sympathetically the frustrations that the Council members and officers must have experienced in those early years. A Select Committee of the House of Commons set up in 1904 to consider the state registration of nurses reported in 1905; one of its recommendations was:

> Your Committee are agreed that it is desirable that a Register of Nurses should be kept by a Central Body appointed by the State and that, while it is not desirable to prohibit unregistered persons from nursing for gain, no person should be entitled to assume the designation of 'Registered Nurse' whose name is not upon the Register.

This became a feature of the Nurses Registration Act of 1919, which also contained the means whereby those persons who had previously trained as nurses could be admitted to the Register of Nurses when it was opened.

The somewhat anomalous position therefore existed whereby a person could be admitted to the Register of Nurses by virtue of a training prior to 1925, could be removed from the Register of Nurses for some misdemeanour, and could then continue legally to practise nursing for gain provided she or he did not claim to be a state registered nurse. This is exactly what happened in respect of only the second person to be removed from the Register. For the young Council it must have been frustration enough, but the matter was compounded over several years by the fact that the lady was the subject of many reports for her misdeeds, and the Council could do nothing about it!

SUGGESTED FURTHER READING

Bendall E. R. D. & Raybould E. (1969) *A History of the General Nursing Council for England and Wales, 1919–1969*. London: H. K. Lewis.
Hector W. (1973) *Mrs Bedford Fenwick and the Rise of Professional Nursing*. London: Royal College of Nursing.
Abel-Smith B. (1960) *The History of the Nursing Profession*. London: Heinemann (reprinted in paperback 1979).

4

The Framework of Professional
Nursing Discipline

Membership of a profession, in matters of nursing ethics and conduct, involves the judgement of a nurse by his or her professional peers. This is essential if any claim by nursing and nurses to the word *profession* is to be sustained.

The responsibility for operating the system by which complaints against registered or enrolled nurses are investigated and considered, and for constantly appraising the efficiency and effectiveness of that system, lies with the same statutory bodies to which Parliament has given the responsibility for controlling admission to the Register and Roll of Nurses in the United Kingdom (i.e., the General Nursing Council for England and Wales, the General Nursing Council for Scotland, and the Northern Ireland Council for Nurses and Midwives). The legislation previously described was designed for the protection of the public to be carried out by these representatives of the nursing profession with appropriate support from selected and appointed representatives of other professions and from those who could fairly be said to represent the public interest. The main functions of the nursing statutory bodies are illustrated in Figure 1. The nature of professional responsibility and the wording of the legislation that established and sustains those statutory bodies places 'the public' in the centre and their functions around them. The public should expect nurses to have achieved an appropriate degree of proven competence before admission to the Register or Roll (section A, Fig. 1); accessible records for verification of that competence (section B, Fig. 1); and appropriate consideration if that competence is in question (section C, Fig. 1). My emphasis is on the responsibility contained in section C. To appreciate satisfactorily how this responsibility is fulfilled let us look at the structure of the statutory bodies concerned.

The membership and structure of the General Nursing Council for England and Wales (Fig. 2) provides an acceptable example. Although there are differences in the respective Acts of Parliament and Statutory Rules, similar principles apply to the other bodies concerned with this subject in the United Kingdom. Of the forty-two members of Council, the law requires that at least twenty-eight must be nurses who, at the time of their election or appointment, must be in current practice. The 5-year terms for elected and appointed members commence in different years.

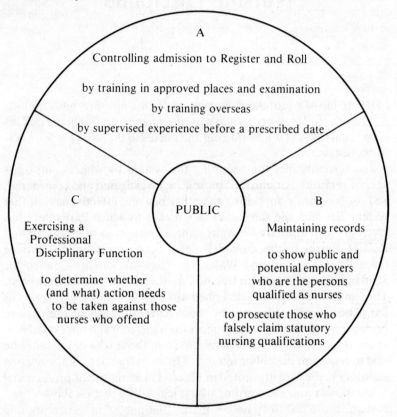

FIGURE 1. The main functions of the nursing statutory bodies.

The membership of various committees is determined in accordance with current legislation. At the September meeting of Council which ends one year and opens a new year the members appoint or elect from within their own number those who will serve on the various committees for the year commencing in October. In practice members are invited to offer their services for membership of particular committees (being first made aware of the subject matter dealt with and the time commitment involved), after which a ballot is held where the offers exceed the number of places.

The two committees of the General Nursing Council for England and Wales with responsibility for professional discipline are the Investigating and Disciplinary Committees. There are a number of respects in which they differ from the remainder; these are:

a. While a member of Council can be a member of any other permutation of committees the law does not allow membership of both the Investigating Committee (eight members) and the Disciplinary

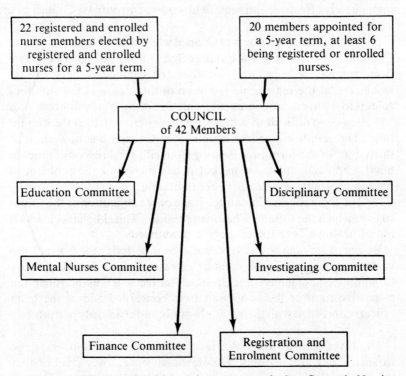

FIGURE 2. The membership and structure of the General Nursing Council for England and Wales.

Committee (sixteen members from January, 1981). This is eminently sensible law, in that it ensures that any case of alleged professional misconduct that reaches the Disciplinary Committee (the only committee able to remove from a nurse the right to practice in his or her chosen profession) will have been the subject of consideration by two entirely separate groups of members constituting more than half the Council.

b. With the exception of the Investigating and Disciplinary Committees, the committees of the Council must operate (in respect of those policies they wish to change or introduce) by bringing recommendations to the Council meeting where they can be debated, and those recommendations either rejected or accepted with or without amendment. This is not the case with the two committees which here concern us. They deal almost entirely with matters concerning individual nurses, and they simply report to Council what they have already done in accordance with the power and responsibility placed upon them in law. Their decisions concerning individual nurses are immediately effective, and require no endorsement from Council as a whole.

c. Of the sixteen members of Council who make up the Disciplinary Committee the existing law requires that at least two must be drawn from among the non-nurse members of Council. I have always assumed that the reasonable intention of this clause in the statutory rules is to try to ensure some representation of consumer interest. This has often been difficult to achieve, but never more than at the present time. The number of nurse members of Council has now risen to thirty-four of the forty-two. Bearing Council's total responsibilities in mind I applaud this position, but it has increased the problem of finding appropriate consumer representation.

d. The Disciplinary Committee is the only Committee of the Council over which the Council Chairman presides. This, I believe, marks it out as having a very special degree of authority.

Before examining how cases come to be reported to the Council, the various types of case, the conduct of cases before the Disciplinary Committee, and many other related subjects, let us consider the respective roles of the two committees concerned and of the main officers concerned with their being lawfully and efficiently performed.

The Investigating Committee is composed of eight members of the Council. They are, in effect, a professional sieve. They meet neither the person who is the subject of a case nor any complainants. Instead, they receive and carefully study a set of documents in respect of each case, and then they come together for a monthly meeting to arrive at collective professional judgements. The options open to them in respect of the various categories of case are:

1. *Where the case involves a qualified nurse who has been found guilty of a criminal offence* which has subsequently been reported to the Council, the Investigating Committee can decide that the matters reported:

a. are of no concern to the Council *or*

b. are of concern to the Council (by which they effectively label the matter as professional misconduct), but that some words of caution and guidance conveyed by letter will suffice *or*

c. justify a hearing before the Disciplinary Committee.

2. *Where the case involves a qualified nurse against whom allegations of professional misconduct have been received* the Investigating Committee can:

a. decline to proceed with the case *or*

b. forward the case for inquiry before the Disciplinary Committee *or*

c. where the allegations are admitted in writing, but are not considered sufficiently serious to justify a hearing before the Disciplinary Committee, decide that the matters reported are of concern to the Council (thus labelling them as professional misconduct), but that some words of caution and guidance conveyed by letter will suffice.

3. *Where the case involves a student or pupil nurse whose training has not been discontinued* as a result of an incident reported to the Council the Investigating Committee can:

a. decide that the nurse's examination entry, when eventually submitted, will be accepted provided that no other offence is committed in the meantime *or*

b. decide that they wish to consider the matter again when an application for examination entry is eventually submitted with its indication of support from the director of nurse education *or*

c. decline to accept an application for entry to an examination, as a result of which the applicant must have the opportunity of a personal hearing before the Disciplinary Committee.

4. *Where the case involves a student or pupil nurse whose training has been discontinued* as a result of an incident reported to the Council the Investigating Committee can ban resumption of training. If they do not wish to impose such a ban they must answer the question How much training must this person undergo if he or she is able to obtain a place to resume training? In answering the question before them the Investigating Committee will take account not only of the length of the training already completed and the duration of the break in training but also of the nature of the offence leading to discontinuation and how the person views it in retrospect.

The minimum requirement the Committee can impose is that required by the 'break in training' statutory rules of those who have discontinued training honourably, but they are permitted by existing law to extend that period, even to the point of invalidating all previous training and practical examination success if they think fit. The person whose training has been extended in this way, or who is barred from continuation or resumption, can, if aggrieved by that decision, request a personal hearing before the Disciplinary Committee.

5. *Where the case involves a person who has been found guilty of a criminal offence, or against whom allegations of misconduct have been made subsequent to a supported examination entry being submitted but before registration or enrolment*, the Investigating Committee must consider the matter when that person applies for admission to the Register or Roll of Nurses. Having considered all the facts they may accept the entry (while expressing some words of admonition if they think fit), but if they feel unable so to do the matter must be referred to the Disciplinary Committee for a hearing.

The Disciplinary Committee is composed of sixteen members of Council, two of whom must not be nurses. In matters of professional discipline theirs is the ultimate power, in that they alone can remove a person from the Register or Roll of Nurses, and that decision (though it can be the subject of an appeal to the High Court) is immediately effective. Unlike the Investigating Committee, this Committee does receive the respondent in person whenever he or she can be persuaded to attend. The options open to them in respect of the various categories of case are:

1. *Where the case involves a qualified nurse who has been found guilty of criminal offence* the guilt is established by presentation of the relevant certified document from the Court confirming that finding. The Disciplinary Committee must then decide if they consider the facts to be misconduct in a professional sense. If they decide that they are then they must hear the available evidence in mitigation or aggravation, and must then:

a. administer a caution, but take no further action *or*

b. postpone their judgement on the matter for a stated period, thus leaving the nurse with the right to practise, and providing him or her with an opportunity to prove himself or herself deserving of that trust before a final consideration of their professional status *or*

c. decide to remove the nurse's name from the Register or Roll of Nurses, and thus to make it unlawful for them to work in or apply for any post for which a statutory nursing qualification is required.

(Appeal to the High Court is available for category C only.)

2. *Where the case involves a qualified nurse against whom allegations of misconduct have been made* (and assuming it has not been rendered unnecessary by a written admission to the allegations made by the nurse after receiving the notice of the enquiry before the Disciplinary Committee), the Committee must first hear evidence in

support of the allegations and in rebuttal, and must then decide whether, in their collective view, the allegations have been proved beyond reasonable doubt. If the Committee consider the allegations (or at least some of them) proved they must then decide whether they consider the now proven facts to be misconduct in a professional sense. If they decide that the matters are professional misconduct they must hear any available evidence in mitigation or aggravation and then choose from the available decisions referred to in paragraph 1.

3. *Where the case involves a qualified nurse previously placed on postponed judgement, and now returning for the resumed hearing*, the Disciplinary Committee have available to them exactly the same range of decisions as referred to in paragraphs 1 and 2 for 'first' hearings.

4. *Where the case involves a discontinued student or pupil nurse whose training has been extended or who has been barred from resuming training*, the Disciplinary Committee can either endorse the Investigating Committee's decision or (in the light of the evidence presented) amend that decision. Such a hearing sometimes results in the Disciplinary Committee further extending the residue of training about which the applicant was already aggrieved.

There is no appeal against their decision, but the person who is barred from resuming training may subsequently apply for that barrier to be removed.

5. *Where the case involves a student or pupil nurse whose application for entry to a Council examination has not been accepted by the Investigating Committee* the Disciplinary Committee must decide to accept or reject the application.

There is no appeal against their decision.

6. *Where the case involves a former student or pupil nurse who has passed the required examinations and completed the statutory training*, but whose application for admission to the Register or Roll of Nurses the Investigating Committee have not felt able to accept, the Disciplinary Committee must decide to accept or reject that application.

There is no appeal against their decision.

7. *Where the case involves an application for restoration to the Register or Roll of Nurses* from which the applicant had previously been removed, the Disciplinary Committee must decide to accept or reject the application.

There is no appeal against a decision to reject an application for restoration.

That fairly basic explanation of the roles of the two committees in respect of the various types of case draws attention at once to the awesome power of each group of members, and to the limitations imposed upon them.

For the Investigating Committee the limitation on their power in respect of qualified nurses lies in that the most that they can do is to decide that a set of facts or allegations 'justify a hearing before the Disciplinary Committee'. They have no power to make recommendations to the Disciplinary Committee as to their subsequent judgement. If they are limited, however, in that respect (I believe quite rightly) their power over the same category of nurses is still awesome as they are able to prevent the Disciplinary Committee from considering all those cases in which they (the Investigating Committee) choose not to proceed, or deem it appropriate only to caution and counsel by letter. Even the Council as a whole have no power in law to overrule them.

That same awesome power of the Investigating Committee is the major limitation on the Disciplinary Committee's power. They can deal only with those qualified nurse cases that the Investigating Committee refer to them. Their power lies in their authority to remove nurses from the Register or Roll, to reject applications for examination entry or for registration or enrolment, and to reject applications for restoration to the Register or Roll. There is a right of appeal (to the High Court) only in removal from the Register or Roll, but meantime (probably many months) their decision stands. Their decision to remove a nurse from the Register or Roll is immediately effective.

The reader will appreciate that this responsibility is heavy to bear and will recognise from the explanation (and the statistics presented in Appendix C to indicate the volume and range of the cases presenting in a fairly typical year) that the nursing profession as a whole owe a considerable debt to their few colleagues who have, over the years, borne the burden of this work.

Before the committees can meet and turn their attention to the matters requiring the members' collective consideration and judgement a substantial amount of work must be performed, largely unseen, by a number of people. All this is directed towards the moment when the officials directly concerned with the conduct of the meetings play their parts in assisting the committees to function in such a way that appropriate and just consideration of the matters before them is possible.

The first of the officials concerned (as the system is operated by the General Nursing Council for England and Wales) is the deputy registrar. The staff of the disciplinary section work in a line relationship to him or her in accordance with the procedures described in Chapter 5. Suffice it here to say that, in respect of the committees, it is the deputy registrar's task to ensure that

all appropriate documents are assembled and placed before them
no inadmissable evidence is included in those documents
a quorum of members is available

Disciplinary Committee timetables are prepared that recognise the travelling problems of committee members, respondents and witnesses

all relevant support services are available

the committee's decisions are properly recorded and acted upon without delay

The wider role of the Council's solicitor is detailed in Chapters 5 and 6. His or her role in direct respect of the Investigating Committee is primarily one of assistance with the assembly of relevant information, and advising the Committee on the viability of evidence in allegation cases.

The third of the officials seen by any members of the public who choose to attend the Disciplinary Committee is the legal assessor. Such a participative representative of the law has been required by the statutory rules since 1961. The rules require that whenever the Disciplinary Committee are sitting to hear cases (whether those cases arise out of criminal convictions or allegations of misconduct) they must be accompanied by a legal assessor who must be 'a barrister, advocate or solicitor of not less than 10 years' standing'.

At a meeting of the Disciplinary Committee of the General Nursing Council for England and Wales in 1979 the Chairman, Zena Oxlade, made a statement in public which reminded the committee members, the staff, and the members of the public in attendance of the purpose of the committee and the role within its proceedings of the legal assessor. It explains the legal assessor's role and aptly rounds off the framework of Professional Discipline today.

> It is useful from time to time to refresh our minds about the objects of this Committee and how those objects are to be achieved.
> The cases which are referred to us fall into one of two categories—allegation cases and conviction cases. Today we consider only allegation cases.
> We are here to consider two cases referred to us for inquiry by the Investigating Committee. The fact that a case has been referred to us does not mean necessarily either that the facts alleged against a nurse are true or that his or her name should be removed from the Register. All the Investigating Committee have done is to decide that if the allegations made against a respondent are true there is a need, in the public interest, to consider whether he or she should be permitted to continue to practise nursing.
> In an allegation case the respondent is charged with being guilty of misconduct in relation to certain facts alleged against him or her in

the charge. When both parties have completed their case the Committee goes into camera to decide whether, on the evidence adduced, the facts alleged are proved and then, if they are, whether they constitute misconduct in a professional respect.

In deciding whether the facts alleged are proved we should bear in mind that the standard of evidence required in a case before the Committee has always been held to be similar to that required in a criminal court—that is to say, that the Committee must believe the facts to have been proved beyond reasonable doubt. It is not enough for us to think it probable that the facts alleged are true; we must have no reasonable doubt about them.

If the facts are found to be proved we have to consider whether they amount to 'misconduct in a professional respect'. It is for this Committee only to decide whether a particular action of a particular nurse amounts to professional misconduct. In reaching a decision each member may ask himself [or herself] the questions 'Have the actions of the respondent damaged the public's confidence in the profession as a whole?' 'Have the actions of the respondent resulted in actual or potential harm to any members of the vulnerable public?' If the answer is 'yes', then they may well decide to consider it professional misconduct.

The Committee must exclude from its mind any evidence which is not submitted at the time of the hearing. It is for this reason Committee members have only the Charge and no other papers. The reason for this is that, in fairness to a respondent, it must be possible for him or her, directly or through a representative, to challenge that evidence. And finally on the question of evidence the legal adviser will help us if the admissibility of evidence is challenged. The legal assessor is not here to advise us other than on points of law. He is only here to ensure that our procedure is correct in accordance with the rules and in accordance with accepted legal procedure and to advise us on the admissibility of evidence.

5

Into the Professional Sieve

The relevant clause of the Nurses Act, 1957, which provides the basis of the professional disciplinary process in nursing to be operated by the General Nursing Council for England and Wales is found in Section 7 of that Act, and the key parts read:

> The Council shall make rules prescribing:
> a. the causes for which, the conditions under which and the manner in which persons may be removed from the Register and the Roll respectively; and
> b. the procedure for, and the fee to be payable on, the restoration to the Register and the Roll respectively of persons who have been removed therefrom.
> A person aggrieved by the removal of his [or her] name from the Register or Roll may, within three months after the date on which notice is given . . . by the appropriate authority that his [or her] name has been so removed, appeal against the removal to the High Court, and on any such appeal the High Court may give such directions in the matter as it thinks proper, including directions as to the costs of the appeal, and the order of the High Court shall be final.

The equivalent section of the Nurses, Midwives and Health Visitors Act is quoted and discussed in Chapter 9.

While that piece of text provides the basis, the system that is operated has also to be defined legally in some detail. This detail is to be found (in respect of registered nurses) in The Nurses Rules Approval Instrument, 1969 (Statutory Instrument 1969 No. 1675), and the Enrolled Nurses Rules Approval Instrument, 1969 (Statutory Instrument No. 1674). In the former the relevant section is the long sequence of rules commencing at Rule 42. In the latter the relevant section is the long sequence of rules commencing at Rule 37. Apart from the fact that in one place the words *registered* and *Register* are used, and in the other *enrolled* and *Roll* the two rules commencing these sequences are the same.

39

The opening words of the Rules 42 and 37 are important to any consideration of the professional disciplinary process, since they immediately draw attention to the things that the Council are required by law to consider. Both rules begin:

> When it is brought to the notice of the Council that a registered [or enrolled] nurse has been convicted of a crime, or where she [or he] is alleged to have been guilty of any misconduct during the period in which her [or his] name is in the Register [or Roll].

That brief extract immediately points to the fact that there are two starting points. The first concerns those registered and enrolled nurses who are found guilty in criminal courts; the second, those who are the subject of complaints that allege misconduct. Though that extract may be very brief it nonetheless contains several extremely significant points which require closer consideration before moving on to how the process (devised under the terms of the law in the form of the Statutory Rules) operates. I must emphasise that the rules *do not*:

a. define the nature of the 'crimes' that are considered deserving of report (this is administratively determined in a way described and commented on later in this chapter)

b. limit the sources of 'allegations' to employers or other professional nurses, thus allowing any citizen the right to complain about any nurse with the knowledge that the law will then require the allegations to be investigated. (Some case histories in Appendix A provide examples of allegations brought against nurses by people exercising their right as citizens)

c. limit the Council's concern (or its ability and responsibility to take action) to those cases where the registered or enrolled nurse is in employment at the time that he or she is found guilty in court or is the subject of allegations, or those incidents which occurred in the course of his or her nursing duties.

The first part of the professional disciplinary process as operated by the General Nursing Council for England and Wales in accordance with the nurses and enrolled nurses rules, is illustrated in Figure 3. Let us examine the two sources of reports—'findings of guilt' and 'allegations'—for a clearer understanding of the subsequent stages of the process.

Dealing first with those cases that result from the establishment of guilt in criminal courts, you will notice that Figure 3 indicates that the police make reports to the Council. In doing so they are simply acting in accordance with a Home Office instruction to the various police forces. They are required to report relevant findings of guilt of both qualified nurses and those in training for a statutory qualification. The broad criteria set out in the circular require that categories of offences reported should be those involving drugs, violence, dishonesty, indecency, and excessive alcohol abuse, since these things may (not must)

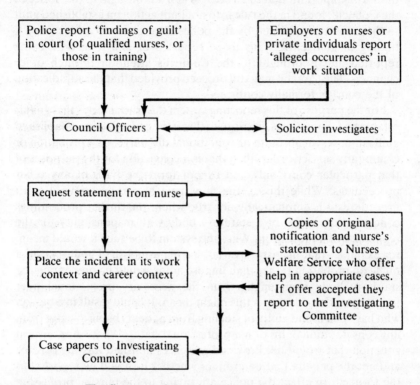

FIGURE 3. The first part of the professional disciplinary process.

reflect on a person's suitability to continue in his or her profession. The general (and I believe totally reasonable) philosophy behind this practice is that policemen, magistrates, or even judges cannot properly determine what is of concern to a particular profession, but rather that such matters should be considered and determined by a group of members of that profession sitting in collective professional judgement. This seems to me a right and proper basis for a reporting system which initiates a process of professional peer judgement, since it has allowed the nursing profession to determine and state the broad categories of offence in which it has an interest, thus removing from the police the onus of deciding what may be of concern to the nursing profession.

For the most part the system works well, but inevitably some findings of guilt that should be reported by the police are overlooked. It is therefore important that the words 'When it is brought to the notice of the Council', found in the rules, do not limit action on established guilt to those matters reported by the police. There are occasions when a finding of guilt either fails to be reported or is a long time being reported and is brought to the Council's attention through other channels. The Council may still proceed provided that the adjudication of the court is formally confirmed.

For the purpose of this reporting system the crucial fact is that guilt is established. Sometimes, it is argued that if the court (having established guilt) imposes an absolute or conditional discharge, or a probation or community service order, then that is a conviction for the purposes of that particular court only and cannot form the basis of any other proceedings. While this is true in respect of certain criminal court procedures it is emphatically not true where the further proceedings concerned are those of a statutory body with responsibility for the regulation of a profession. Were the system to be such it would mean, for example, that magistrates who, having established guilt, placed a nurse on probation rather than impose a fine would be preventing the statutory body from engaging in the necessary professional peer judgement. Consider what this might mean. It could result in a person who has been found guilty of stealing from patients being exempt from any consideration of his or her professional status. What a nonsensical situation that would be. Provided guilt is established it is the offence and not the penalty that determines whether it should be reported to the Council. In effect the police are saying to the nursing profession 'There you are, you wanted to know about these things. Now you decide which of them are of concern to your profession'.

The second source of reports, 'allegations', emerges when employers of nurses or private individuals report incidents which they allege to have occurred in a particular nurse's working situation, and which (in the view of the person reporting) warrant some consideration of that nurse's appropriateness to continue in his or her profession. It is my experience that while a majority of such allegations are received from senior nurses (e.g., district or divisional nursing officers), a significant number come from other employees of the specific hospital or location, and a small but seemingly increasing number from private individuals who just chanced to be in the vicinity and were disturbed by what they observed. Case 9 provides an example of the last source of reports.

CASE 9

On a winter evening two young women went to visit a patient (the uncle of one of them) in a geriatric ward. While there they saw a pupil nurse treating another patient in a manner they regarded as reprehensible.

The incident as they subsequently described it concerned a situation wherein the patient concerned was sitting at a long table near to one end of the ward with his back towards the television set. The nurse involved sat almost opposite him, looking past him to watch the programme on television. Of the two other nurses on duty a student nurse was administering medicines, while the other (an SEN) was writing up Kardex notes at the other end of the long table.

The visitors said that the patient could not communicate properly, and muttered for much of the time, sometimes quite loudly. They said that the pupil nurse seemed annoyed that the patient's muttering was interfering with her television watching, and told him quite loudly and curtly to 'shut up'. That having failed, it was said that she repeated the order, but also slapped the patient hard on his hands which were on the table, and that when that also failed she kicked him on the shins beneath the table sufficiently hard for him to cry out in pain.

Having seen and heard all this, the visitors remonstrated with the pupil nurse concerned, but were told that it was none of their business. They then complained to the nurse in charge of the ward, but the response indicated neither concern nor any intention to take action on their complaint. They decided that, if such were the attitudes on the ward, there seemed little point in complaining to the management of that hospital.

When they left the hospital they were very angry and concerned at what they had seen, and convinced each other that they could not simply ignore the matter. They therefore went to the reference section of the nearby Public Library and sought information as to how the nursing profession is regulated. Having found the information they were seeking, they telephoned the General Nursing Council for England and Wales the next morning, and having had their view that it was their right to bring a complaint confirmed, they then submitted their complaint in writing. Their evidence stood up well at the Disciplinary Committee hearing.

In effect, it is any citizen's right, therefore, to complain about any nurse, and in this respect the nurse manager's right is no greater nor is it any less than that of the visitor to a hospital ward. Where such complaints are received it is then incumbent on the Council to have those complaints investigated, because such is the law.

No nurse can have his or her name removed from the Register or Roll of Nurses, and thus be prevented from practising, on the basis of someone else's unproven statements. Those allegations must be thoroughly investigated and tested, no matter what cost in time or money. Furthermore, should the matter be forwarded to the Disciplinary Committee for a hearing, the complainants and any other witnesses to an incident are required to attend to give their evidence, to be cross-examined by the nurse either directly or through a representative, and to be questioned by the members of the Disciplinary Committee. These aspects are more fully described under the role and procedure of the Disciplinary Committee (see Chapter 6). Many of what I call 'allegation' cases never reach that stage.

Is it possible, then, to summarise the types of offence that can be reported? The answer has to be No. Earlier in this chapter I refer to the general categories of offence that the police are required to report (drugs, violence, dishonesty, indecency, and excessive alcohol abuse); each category contains many different types of offence varying in both severity and apparent professional significance. As the pattern of our life in society changes so do the crimes people commit, and while I could produce a detailed list of the offences reported by the police in, say, 1979 it would be no better as a guide for the future than the preceding brief and general criteria. Much the same can be said of allegation cases. The statistics available up to 1978–79 show the continued and growing presence of offences that have to do with drugs (misappropriation, false entries or forgeries in registers, fictitious prescriptions) and the physical abuse of patients. To them, however, has been added an increased number of reports that arise from (a) unfitness on duty due to alcohol and (b) the administration of either unprescribed drugs or excessive doses of prescribed drugs.

Perhaps more significant still is the increase in the number of cases that are directly concerned with nursing practice, where the complainants feel that, by their actions or inactions, the nurses concerned were culpable in a way that might be considered professional misconduct. One such example was contained in case 3 (Chapter 1) where the offence was tantamount to negligence, but some others are more concerned with incompetence. Complainants now seem willing to make a formal accusation about failure to use professional knowledge or exercise professional judgement (where that failure has actual or potential serious consequences) in a way that seems not to have been a feature of the past. There are those who argue that to be short of either knowledge or competence is not misconduct. To me that is only consistent with holding the view that the acquisition of knowledge and competence ceased on the last day of a statutory training period. Surely the public are entitled to expect more from the SRN who has 12 years' postregistration experience than from the SEN who qualified yesterday. Provided such matters are considered in their work and career context the judgements made by other professional nurses on such matters will be fair and just.

A new trend in reports concerns those who by absenting themselves from their duties without good reason are alleged to have put the health, safety or welfare of their patients at risk.

The fields for complaints are wide so a machinery wherein those complaints can be thoroughly tested to assess first guilt and then, if guilt is established, professional gravity is essential.

The notification of a finding of guilt (with other supportive information such as police reports, probation officer's and psychiatrist's reports to courts) or the assembly of the documentary evidence in support of an allegation provides the Council with one side of the story. Obviously, however, no fair and reasonable decision can be made by any Investigating Committee, no matter how wise its members, without knowledge of the work and career context of the incident and of any explanation or, in allegation cases, denial that the nurse concerned may wish to offer.

Let us examine further Figure 3 and the sequence of events that are followed by the General Nursing Council for England and Wales to equip the Investigating Committee to make fair and reasonable decisions. A key point to note is that the nurse is contacted by a letter sent by recorded delivery, told that the finding of guilt has been reported by the police or allegations made against him or her, and asked for any statement, explanation or comments so that the Committee may be as fully informed as possible. I like to believe that the Council would invite such a statement of their own choice were it necessary; as it is, the law in the form of the statutory rules requires such an action. I believe this to be sound law.

The next vital point to notice is the block which contains the words *Place the incident in its work and career context*. I cannot stress too strongly the importance of this aspect. The decision to do this is not a requirement of law; it is a matter of obvious commonsense.

The final point to note is that section set out to the right which refers to the existence and help available from the Nurses Welfare Service. The role of this service is explained more fully in Chapter 7 (and through some of the case studies in Appendix A), but mentioned here because their early involvement in appropriate cases (where an offer of help and support is accepted) is often useful in putting the case into its context, and drawing attention to any social factors that may have been a cause of stress.

The Investigating Committee members come together, each bringing his or her knowledge, experience, and perhaps prejudices, having read the considerable volume of documents sent to them one week earlier, to fulfil their role as the profession's sieve, and to make collective professional judgements.

6

The Disciplinary Committee Hearing: the Preparation and the Event

The percentage of cases involving qualified nurses that the Investigating Committee have considered as justifying a hearing before the Disciplinary Committee in recent years has been about 32 per cent. The percentage of student or pupil nurse cases is much lower, the types of offence on the whole being trivial or not related to patients or nursing practice or both.

Let us consider how the Disciplinary Committee proceed with those new cases that, in the opinion of the Investigating Committee, justify a hearing, those resumed cases that are reconsidered when a period of postponed judgement comes to term, or when an application for restoration to the Register or Roll is to be heard.

When cases are forwarded by the Investigating Committee for the first time, the manner in which that information is conveyed to the nurse who is to become the respondent is most important. If the respondent is a qualified nurse whose suitability to possess the right to practice is to be questioned, two letters are sent by the deputy registrar. The first is the formal Notice of Enquiry letter which must by law be sent with at least 21 days' notice of the hearing, and in exactly the form of words prescribed in the statutory rules. The letter reads:

Disciplinary Committee Nurses Acts 1957 to 1969
Take notice that the charge against you, particulars of which are set forth below, has been brought to the notice of the Council, and that the Disciplinary Committee of the Council propose to investigate such charge at a meeting to be held at the offices of the Council, 23 Portland Place, London W1A 1BA, at   [*time/date*]   and to decide what disciplinary action, if any, should be taken.

Particulars of charge
You are hereby required to attend before the Disciplinary Committee of the Council at the time and place mentioned above and to answer such charge, bringing with you all papers and documents in

47

your possession relevant to the matter and any persons whose
evidence you wish to lay before the Disciplinary Committee.
The following points should be carefully noted:

(a) You are entitled to be represented at the hearing before the
Disciplinary Committee by a friend, or by Counsel or a Solicitor, but
if you propose to employ Counsel or a Solicitor, you should give
written notice to the Registrar at the address mentioned above at
least seven days before the hearing.

(b) You should bring with you to the hearing your certificate of
registration and badge.

Your attention is directed to Part VII of the Nurses Rules, 1969 [or
Enrolled Nurses Rules, 1969], a copy of which is enclosed.

Until the 1976 rule amendments the phrase 'determine whether
your name should be removed from the Register' stood at the end of
the first paragraph where it now reads 'decide what disciplinary action,
if any, should be taken'. I am sure that the previous form led many
people to the conclusion that removal was inevitable, and as a consequence led to the frequent absence of the respondents. This is now
largely remedied.

In practice, if there will be a significant delay between the Investigating Committee decision and the case being scheduled for hearing on a
particular day, a brief letter is sent to the nurse to advise him or her that
the case has been forwarded for a Disciplinary Committee hearing, but
that it is not yet possible to give precise information as to the date on
which it will be heard. This enables the nurse to take steps concerning
the preparation of his or her case to put to the Committee.

The second letter that the Council's officers send is not required by
law, but is sent so that the respondent nurse is fully informed about his
or her rights of attendance, representation, and the like. The text of
this covering letter has changed over the years. In early 1980 there
were two versions—one each for the conviction and allegation cases,
respectively.

Conviction case letter

Dear

Your letter submitting a statement was brought to the attention of
the Investigating Committee of the Council at its recent meeting.
After careful consideration, it was decided that this matter justified a
hearing before the Disciplinary Committee. I am therefore enclosing
a formal notice of the hearing of your case by that Committee.
The Committee would be willing to receive letters from your
employer or any other persons which you may consider helpful to
your case. In addition you may submit medical evidence regarding
your health at the time of the incident if you wish. If you intend to be

legally represented, your Counsel or Solicitor will presumably put forward any medical or other evidence you may desire. If you do not intend to be legally represented but wish to submit medical evidence, you should either ask the doctor concerned (if he or she cannot attend in person) to write direct to the Council before the hearing, or you should yourself send or bring with you to the hearing a letter from the doctor.

You might also find it helpful to seek the advice of any professional or other organisation. If you are a member of a Trade Union and intend that they will assist and represent you at the hearing, you must inform them of the date and time of the hearing of your case without delay.

I must emphasise that you do not have to attend the meeting if you would prefer not to, but the Committee members would obviously find it helpful if you are able.

I must also emphasise that the matter has not been pre-judged, and the Committee really do want to understand the incident fully. If you are able to attend the hearing, travelling expenses at second class rail fare rate (or the equivalent if you did not travel by rail) will be paid to you in cash at these offices.

I hope that this information will be helpful to you in the preparation of your case, but if you are not clear on any point please do not hesitate to let me know.

Yours sincerely,

Allegation case letter

Dear

Your letter submitting a statement was brought to the attention of the Investigating Committee of the Council at its recent meeting. After careful consideration, it was decided that this matter justified a hearing before the Disciplinary Committee. I am, therefore, enclosing a formal notice of the hearing of your case by that Committee.

If it is your intention to admit the allegations in the Charge, it will be very helpful if you would write to me to this effect as soon as possible. This may enable me to cancel the attendance of the witnesses. It is, of course, entirely for you to decide whether or not to admit the allegations, and if you intend to be represented by Counsel or a Solicitor or to seek advice of any professional or other organisation. If you are a member of a Trade Union and intend that they will assist and represent you at the hearing, you must inform them of the date and time of the hearing of your case without delay.

Whether or not you wish to deny the allegations, you do not have to attend the meeting if you prefer not to, but I strongly advise it. If you will be denying the allegations it will obviously be in your best interests to attend to present your case either yourself or through your representative. If you will be admitting the allegations, the Committee members will still find it helpful if you come and you can then, of course, give your account of the incident.

Whatever you decide, it will be very helpful if you will write to me and indicate whether you intend to come to the hearing.

I must emphasise that the matter has not been pre-judged, and the Committee really do want to understand the incident fully. If you are able to attend the hearing, travelling expenses at second class rail fare rate (or the equivalent if you did not travel by rail) will be paid to you in cash at these offices.

The Committee would be willing to receive letters from your employer or any other persons which you may consider helpful to you. In addition, you may, if you wish, submit medical evidence regarding your health at the time of the incident. If you intend to be represented, your representative will no doubt produce any references or medical reports you wish to put forward. If you do not intend to be represented, but wish to submit medical evidence, you should either ask the doctor concerned (if he or she cannot attend in person) to write direct to the Council before the hearing, or you should send or bring with you to the hearing a letter from the doctor.

I hope that this information will be helpful to you in the preparation of your case, but if you are not clear on any point please contact me.

Yours sincerely,

The sending of those letters to the registered or enrolled nurses concerned therefore gives them not only precise information on the date and time of the hearing but considerable additional information which should help them to both understand their position and prepare thoughtfully for the hearing. It is not intended that those letters should preempt any further questions, but rather leave the channels of communication open so that the supplementary questions specific to an individual case may be asked.

The period between sending the Notice of Enquiry and covering letters and the actual date of the hearings tends to be very active, with many questions asked and answers given. It is in this period, when the nurse respondent knows that his or her qualification is in jeopardy, that he or she is more likely than before (either directly or through his or her appointed representative) to speak to the officers about the possible outcome, to discuss problems about arranging representation, and to establish contact with the Nurses Welfare Service if that has not already been done.

Another book would be necessary if the many and various types of questions that are asked and the answers given in this period were to be listed. There is one question, however, that is asked so frequently that it would be remiss of me not to mention it here. It comes from those nurses who have been summoned to appear before the Disciplinary Committee, but who are not members of any professional association or trade union, and are doubtful if they can meet the cost of legal representation. They call in, write or telephone (sometimes sounding somewhat despairing, and feeling that all is lost). They are told that

a. their attendance is of the utmost importance, and that the Committee will really want to meet them and to hear from them before making their decision

b. while representation is desirable it is not essential, since the Committee members' questions will form a basis for an unrepresented respondent to explain the circumstances of the incident(s), and the legal assessor will guide him or her in the questioning of witnesses *and*

c. while legal aid is not available for a hearing of the Disciplinary Committee, it is possible (under the terms of the Legal Advice and Assistance Act, 1972) to obtain the services of a solicitor free of charge (subject to certain conditions) to prepare a written submission to assist them to represent themselves before the Committee.

This supplementary information, when considered with the guidance, contained in the letters, frequently results in nurse respondents attending, even though unrepresented.

So much for the work that is involved in calling an individual respondent to attend on a given date. I am confident that the reader will readily appreciate that a considerable logistical problem has to be tackled before the Notice of Enquiry letters can be sent, and a number of others in the period between dispatch of those letters and the actual meeting.

First, an agenda must be constructed for the day's meeting from the cases forwarded for hearings by the Investigating Committee. (With the General Nursing Council for England and Wales the position is usually that, at any given time, the accumulated forwarded cases require approximately 30 hours of Committee time.) In constructing such an agenda the officer concerned must:

a. assess the likely duration of each case to be included

b. allocate each case to a time of day that will allow the respondent and all others involved to travel from and return to their homes, *or* indicate that a case has been called for a time which will involve an overnight stay, and offer to arrange accommodation *and*

c. ensure that all the required witnesses, police officers, (etc.) are available, and instruct the solicitor to subpoena any essential participants who seem reluctant to attend

That having been done, attention must be turned to arranging or confirming the attendance of all other key participants whose presence is essential. The check list includes:

i. Have we a quorum of Disciplinary Committee members available, plus at least one to spare in case of illness? (Obviously cases would not be called for a date when the general response of committee members had indicated that a quorum was not available, but other commitments in the members' professional working lives can emerge to change the earlier prediction.)

ii. Have we avoided the unacceptable match of a committee member and a nurse respondent from the same area (or otherwise known to each other), and if not do we have an attendance of members in excess of the quorum figures so that the member in question can stand down for that case?

iii. Have we an appointed legal assessor? If not what other barrister, advocate or solicitor whose experience satisfies the rules is available for appointment for that day?

iv. Is an official shorthand writer available to record and produce verbatim transcripts of all cases?

v. In those cases where the context may be crucial to the decisions, have we invited the appropriate nurse manager to attend or send a representative? (*Invite* is the operative word where the evidence to be given will be heard at the mitigation or aggravation stage of the hearing, rather than be evidence that is concerned with establishing guilt or innocence. Unfortunately some nurse managers who have by then dismissed from employment a nurse who is the subject of a Disciplinary Committee hearing regard it as no longer any of their business and do not attend. This seems to indicate that their concerns are only for their patients at a particular point in time, rather than for patients as a whole, and for the standards of the profession.)

And then in parallel, in terms of time, with all that it is necessary to:

a. prepare the papers that will be sent in advance to members of the Committee (ensuring that they contain nothing 'inadmissible')

b. prepare copies of those papers for the respondent or his or her representative or both

c. prepare copies of other documents which either may be or will be required at the hearings, but which cannot be supplied to members or respondents in advance

d. calculate the likely travelling (etc.) expenses of respondents in order that sufficient money is available to repay those expenses (where information becomes available, usually through the Nurses Welfare Service, that there are financial difficulties that may otherwise prevent attendance a rail ticket is sent in advance)

e. arrange for the repayment of official witnesses expenses *and*

f. continue to respond to or liaise with respondents, solicitors, trade union or professional association representatives, past or present employers, and the press as appropriate

Lest it be thought that the logistical problem is not particularly great I must add that Disciplinary Committee meetings are now so frequent that at least four such cycles are usually overlapping. These are being operated by the group of staff who also have responsibility for the work already described in relation to the Investigating Committee, and who will still have responsibilities in respect of the actual Disciplinary Committee hearings and their aftermath. This is said not as a complaint but a statement of fact. I would not wish it to be otherwise, and I hold the view that to create an atmosphere in which the staff concerned with the cases are not able to maintain contact throughout will only make for a less thorough, less concerned, and less compassionate management of those cases, and almost certainly for conclusions that have been a dangerously long time in the making. (This point which is a comment on the present but with thought for the future is explored further in Chapter 10.)

We move now to the hearing itself. Christine Hancock writes

> To be present as an observer at a GNC Disciplinary Committee
> hearing is an impressive and valuable occasion for any nurse. The
> hearing is conducted with the utmost compassion and professional
> integrity, and every offence is considered in its context.

I like to believe that this is true. It is certainly what the officers of the Council and members of the Disciplinary Committee have strived to achieve over the years. What, then is the setting, and what the procedures that led at least one observer not only to regard them so highly (many others have commented favourably after attendance at the Disciplinary Committee as observers) but to write it down for all to read? First the setting.

The respondent nurse, having been received elsewhere in the building, reassured, paid expenses, and given any additional papers, is also given a diagram of the council room in which the hearing will take place, and is informed about the procedure. The layout of the room into which he or she will step at the appropriate time is shown in Figure 4. The details of the procedure to be followed vary with the type of case. My purpose at this stage is to explain, in general terms, the manner in which the Disciplinary Committee operates in fulfilment of its role.

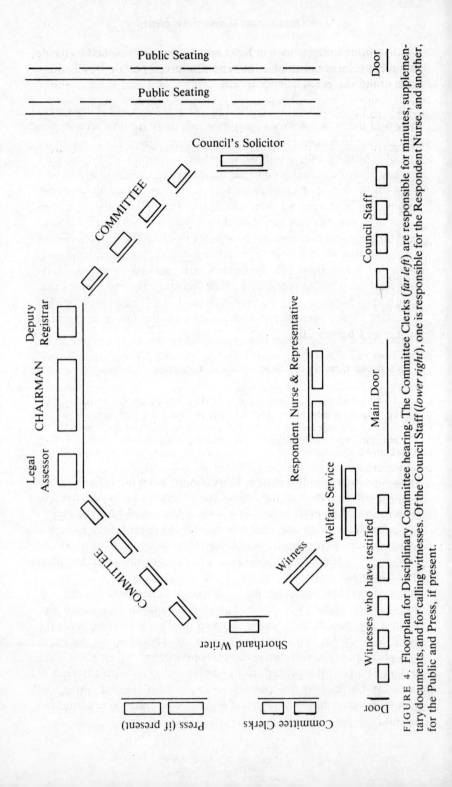

FIGURE 4. Floorplan for Disciplinary Committee hearing. The Committee Clerks (far left) are responsible for minutes, supplementary documents, and for calling witnesses. Of the Council Staff (lower right), one is responsible for the Respondent Nurse, and another, for the Public and Press, if present.

In all cases the chairman will welcome the respondent, and ensure that it is the right person, before the charge is read in new cases, or the details of the previous hearing are recalled in the case of restoration applications or hearings being resumed at the end of periods of postponed judgement.

If the case is the result of a finding of guilt in a criminal court the Committee must accept the court's certificate as proof, and therefore as the baseline from which they must work. It is pointless for a respondent nurse to argue at this stage that he or she was not guilty, even though a plea of guilty was made in court. To plead guilty when you are not is an unwise thing to do, as it can have serious professional ramifications. The Committee must accept the proof of guilt, must decide if the proven facts constitute professional misconduct, and, if they consider those facts to be misconduct, must arrive at an appropriate judgement on the case.

If the case is the result of allegations, then, unless since receiving the Notice of Enquiry summoning the case and setting out the charge the nurse concerned has admitted the allegations in writing, the Committee must first do what in the other type of case the court has already done. They must hear the evidence and decide whether the allegations are proved. If they decide that the allegations have been proved to them beyond reasonable doubt, they must then (as with the conviction type of case) decide whether the proven facts constitute misconduct, and if they decide Yes they must then proceed to make a judgement. Throughout all of this process every effort is made to see the case in its context, and ample opportunity is provided for the respondent nurse to produce evidence of mitigating or extenuating circumstances.

In the preceding paragraphs and in Chapter 4, I refer to *professional misconduct*, or *misconduct in a professional sense*. But what does that mean? Over the years I have addressed audiences (mainly of nurses) throughout Great Britain, and have often been faced by questioners who ask where in nursing law misconduct is defined, and what list of offences constitute misconduct. The answer is (and for nursing I hope will remain) that there is no such definition, and there is no such list.

What, then, is professional misconduct?

The answer: It is what the Committee (primarily composed of nurses), as a collective judgement, decide it is in respect of a particular case, when they have heard all the evidence, and set the case in its context.

Readily I admit that this means there may be some inconsistency, but I would argue that it is the inconsistency of justice rather than injustice. The alternative would be actually to list in the statutory rules those things that would be regarded as professional misconduct. This would be deplorable as it would become impossible to consider an incident in its context before so labelling it, and because such a list would be out of date within weeks of being embodied in law.

By way of illustration let me refer to a case wherein the nurse admitted the allegations made against her, but in the particular quite unsatisfactory circumstances of that case the Disciplinary Committee on the day decided that they did not regard the matter as professional misconduct.

CASE 10

A 40-year-old SRN appeared before the Disciplinary Committee charged with administering unprescribed drugs to patients in her care. The case was unusual, in that she had made no attempt to conceal the fact that the drugs had been administered (written record was made of it in the Kardex records, in the patients' records, and in several other places), and at the Committee she readily admitted that the charge was true.

The incidents had occurred in a cottage hospital in a remote rural setting. The nurse concerned had been approached to assist the nurse managers by covering the maternity leave of the nurse/midwife who normally worked on night duty at this hospital. Obviously the reputation in this district of the nurse (who was the subject of the case) must have been good or the nurse managers would not have approached her. She had last worked as a midwife elsewhere in the district for a period that concluded $2\frac{1}{2}$ years before, but she had not worked as a general nurse for over 12 years, and never in this district. Therefore the hospital in which she was invited to work was new territory to her.

The hospital had some 20 beds for general patients, a small maternity unit, and provided a limited casualty service. The nurse (although out of general nursing for some time) found herself in charge of the hospital from her first night on duty, had no other qualified staff, and had no real introduction or orientation to her work and responsibilities, to the geography of the hospital, or to its policies and procedures. The situation was made worse by the fact that for her first four nights on duty her only support was in the person of a new nursing auxiliary.

The medical cover for this hospital was provided by a number of general practitioners. The nurse quickly discovered that they did not readily respond to her calls at night, and that she frequently found herself administering drugs on a verbal instruction following her description of the symptoms. When that occurred it tended to be both several days and several reminders later before the prescription would be written and signed, during which period the nurse's action in administering the drugs could have been questioned.

It was against that background that, during a period of four consecutive nights, all of which were extremely busy, she administered mild hypnotic drugs to four newly admitted patients, all of whom were regularly taking similar (not exactly the same) hypnotics at home. She readily admitted that she had not telephoned any of the doctors (even in retrospect), but illustrated the pressure of work of these occasions which led her not to fulfil her intentions in that regard. She also explained (a) that (on the basis of the experience of previous nights) she would have been told to do exactly what she had done, and (b) that she had fully and openly recorded the fact of the administration of the drugs.

The local nurse manager observed the recorded evidence of the administration of unprescribed drugs some days later, and the nurse was immediately dismissed, and reported to the Council.

So the Committee must decide in each case whether any particular guilt (whether established in a criminal court or before the Committee) is professional misconduct. If they say No, the case stops. If they say Yes, the Committee members must then proceed to make a judgement on the case, but not until they have heard whatever there is to be said, or studied any documents that are submitted, in either mitigation or aggravation.

Let us now concentrate on new cases involving qualified nurses, since these make up a majority of the cases to be considered. The broad principles that apply to this type of case apply equally to all the others.

The mitigation or aggravation stage of the new case hearing is the stage during which the Committee, having already accepted that guilt has been proved, and having decided that such guilt constitutes misconduct in a professional respect (for the purposes of the nursing profession), must endeavour to set the case in its work and career context before proceeding to make one of the decisions required of them in law. The importance of this stage of the hearing is illustrated in Case 11.

CASE 11

A 50-year-old SRN appeared before the Disciplinary Committee of the General Nursing Council for England and Wales, this following her conviction in a Magistrates Court some weeks earlier for the theft of a large quantity of Distalgesic and DF118 tablets from the hospital in which she had been employed as a ward sister for many years. A member of the hospital pharmacy staff had belatedly noticed that the ward in question seemed to be using far more of the drugs named than was normal for that ward, and that this did not seem to match the prescribing pattern of the medical staff concerned. He informed the chief pharmacist, who in turn spoke to a senior member of the nursing staff. In consequence the senior nursing officer spoke to the police (not to the ward sister), and two police officers came to the ward to speak to the staff. The sister told them immediately that there was no need to speak to anyone else on the ward staff, as she had been taking the drugs for her own use.

Seemingly without even asking her why, her nurse managers dismissed her. She went to the Magistrates Court unsupported, and pleaded guilty to the charge, and was fined the sum of £300 and costs. That picture all looks very black, but what emerged about the work and career context for the Committee to take into account in this case? Basically this. The lady had commenced as a student nurse at this same hospital at the age of 18 years, had successfully completed her training and passed her examinations, had then left to undergo midwifery training elsewhere, but immediately after its completion returned to general nursing at her training hospital, and remained there throught the 27 years that elapsed to the time of her summary dismissal. For many years before that occurrence she had been ward sister of a very demanding ward, dealing primarily with patients with traumatic injuries following road or industrial injuries.

Approximately 6 months before her admission to the police that she had removed the analgesic drugs named, and for her own purposes, the pressure of work on her ward had been extremely heavy; this coincided with both a shortage of nursing staff and considerable staff absence due to sickness. It emerged that at that time she had a recurrence of a chronic low-back problem. She told her nursing officer of her problem, and indicated that she would have to go to see her doctor. To this the nursing officer replied 'Don't do that. We can't do without you! Take something for it'.

Well she did take something for it! She took Distalgesic and DF 118, and the quantity she needed to control the pain steadily grew over the next 6 months. So an unwise response to a foolish suggestion (or was it an order?) from her line manager had resulted in the loss of her job, the shame of a court appearance, a punitive fine, and now an appearance before a Committee of her peers who had the power to remove from her the qualification of which she was proud, and the right to work in her chosen profession.

She assumed (having being harshly dealt with by her employers to whom she had given 30 years of exemplary service and by the Magistrates Court) that she would be further punished by removal from the Register. However, that was not the decision of the Committee. They had before them a woman who, having been dismissed from her employment, had been to her doctor, and with the benefits of the medication and physiotherapy prescribed, and freed from the heavy lifting that had been a regular part of her life, was now well again and not in need of the type of drugs she had been taking. She had quickly taken another training course (having concluded that she would be removed from the Register) and at the time of the hearing was working for the Post Office.

Knowledge of the context is important. Whereas in Case 11 it generated sympathy for and understanding of the respondent nurse, and had a mitigating effect, it will sometimes have quite the reverse effect and aggravate the position. The reader may recognise this in the case studies in Appendix A. The stage between proof of misconduct and arrival at judgement on the case provides an opportunity for the Committee to hear and question people, receive documents, and consider reports that may have a bearing on their subsequent deliberations in camera.

When the Committee makes a judgement their role is not to punish those nurses who appear before them; that is the responsibility of the criminal courts in Britain. Nor is it their role to solve the problems of the nurse managers that may result from either precipitate decisions to dismiss certain nurses from employment or hesitation to dismiss when adequate grounds exist. The Committee's role is first to protect the public, second to maintain the standards of the profession, and third (but very firmly within the context of the preceding points) to create a situation in which the rehabilitation of the individual respondents is made possible. In these respects their role is shared with the Investigating Committee, but to the Disciplinary Committee only falls the ultimate responsibility of deciding whether protection of the public lays upon them the painful duty of removing a person's name from the Register of Nurses.

The options from which the Disciplinary Committee of the General Nursing Council for England and Wales must choose if guilt is established, and then that guilt is considered to be misconduct, are shown in Figure 5. The Committee will accept the option *A* (to administer a caution but take no other disciplinary action) if they consider it appropriate on the day. They will do so only if they are suitably convinced that the respondent nurse has fully realised the significance of the action that led him or her to be before the Committee, has learnt from the experience and clearly will not similarly offend in the future, and is a nurse in whose hands sick people could be placed with confidence.

Option *B* (to postpone their judgement for a stated period of time) is frequently chosen by the Committee. The effect of this is that, having established guilt and considered it to be misconduct, the Committee defer their judgement or sentence on the facts in order to see how the respondent nurse progresses. In announcing this decision the chairman explains to the nurse that this means that his or her name remains on the Register (or Roll) of Nurses, that he or she is eligible to work in or apply for any post for which his or her qualification is required, but that at the end of the period there will be another hearing of the case at which the same three options are available to the Committee, and for which they will require (such is the law) at least two references from people with knowledge of the facts, who have also known the person during the intervening period. To that they can add other requirements (e.g., psychiatric reports, probation officer's report) depending on the situation that existed at the first hearing. All this is confirmed in writing, and the nurse is asked to confirm that he or she understands

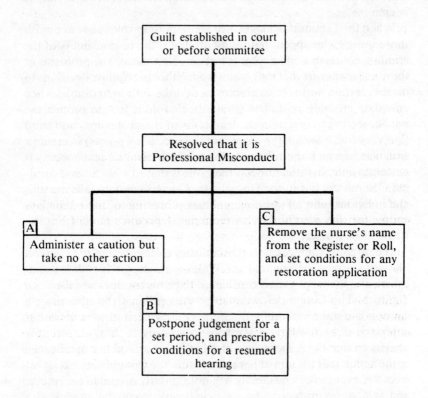

FIGURE 5. The options of the Disciplinary Committee at the stage of judgement.

and will comply with the conditions of postponed judgement. Confirmation and compliance are vital as the statutory rules are such that failure to comply with those conditions (e.g., not nominating referees with knowledge of the facts and who have known the nurse since the first hearing) must result in removal from the Register or Roll.

Option *C* (to remove the name of a nurse from the Register or Roll) is never a pleasant decision for the Committee to have to take and announce, yet it is often necessary if the Committee are to fulfil their role as protectors of the vulnerable public. Earlier I stated that professional discipline is not about punishment, and I adhere to that view even as I write about the removal from people of their right to practise. It is a fact, however, that a majority of those who are removed feel punished on that day, and possibly for some weeks or months afterwards, but many (especially those with drug problems for whom remaining on the Register or Roll would have meant retaining a privileged access to drugs) come to see the day of their removal as the day on which their rehabilitation began. As the influence of the Nurses Welfare Service has grown it has become more common to see respondent nurses before the Disciplinary Committee who, having already established a good and positive relationship with one of the professional social workers, clearly realise that removal is the right decision for them at the particular stage of their life, and see it as a positive contribution to their rehabilitation and the moment at which restoration was set as a target. Those individuals can come at a later date to a restoration hearing feeling that they are going to meet some friends. Whether in the latter category or not, it is certainly not unknown for the individual at a restoration application hearing to thank the Committee for removing him or her from the Register or Roll of Nurses.

The Disciplinary Committee hearing is, and I believe rightly and importantly so, an event conducted in public. It *does* matter that justice should not only be done but be seen to be done. Also an opportunity *must* exist for the public to observe exactly how the nursing profession fulfils this aspect of its responsibility to them. Finally, it *does* provide an opportunity for those members of the profession who choose to attend to share a salutary learning experience, and thus to return to their own work with eyes more alert to the hazards, with a more caring attitude towards their colleagues, and with an enlarged view of professional responsibility. I hope that for those readers who are unable to share that experience the case studies throughout the book will provide something of a challenge.

REFERENCE

Hancock C. (1979) Special industrial relations problems in nursing. In *Industrial Relations in the NHS—the Search for a System*, edited by N. Bosanquet. Tunbridge Wells: Pitman Medical for the King's Fund Centre.

7

The Role of the Nurses Welfare Service

The idea of a welfare service linked to the disciplinary function of a statutory body materialised in 1972 with the setting up of the Nurses Welfare Service. This exciting concept was pioneered by the nursing profession, and the General Nursing Council for England and Wales was the first, and is so far the only, statutory body to have associated such a service with its disciplinary function.

The basic philosophy underlying its establishment was that nursing as a caring profession should be concerned about the relatively small yet significant number of its members who find themselves involved in the disciplinary procedures of the General Nursing Council for England and Wales. It would be all too easy to castigate this group of nurses as the delinquents of the profession who have brought nursing into disrepute by their reprehensible actions. To make such a judgement, however, would be tantamount to an abdication of professional responsibility towards colleagues who often find themselves in this situation because they are sick rather than bad, or are victims of inadequate working environments allowed to exist by those who now reject them.

As a disciplinary case unfolds it so often becomes all too apparent that the nurse concerned has been subjected to intolerable levels of stress, either at home or at work or to a combination of both. The majority of nurses involved are caring, conscientious people with a strong professional commitment.

The 1970s witnessed a fundamental reappraisal of the whole concept of professional discipline on the part of this Council. The subject was discussed at conferences and seminars for nurses throughout the country, resulting in a significant increase in the level of awareness about this important aspect of the Council's work. The Nurses Welfare Service played a vital part in the development of a more caring, positive, enlightened philosophy with regard to professional discipline, in which rehabilitating the nurse concerned became a recognised objective in addition to its fundamental purpose of protecting the vulnerable public from unsafe practitioners.

Having established early in 1972 that it was legally possible to set up the service, the first welfare adviser was appointed in May of that year with the initial task of conducting a survey to identify the needs of nurses who find themselves involved in the disciplinary process of the Council. The production of such a survey involved a detailed study of the legislation governing the Council's disciplinary functions and the underlying professional ethic; attendance at meetings of the Investigating and Disciplinary Committees; a review of past disciplinary cases which illustrated particular areas of need; and an assessment of developing cases to determine the stage at which the need for intervention became evident. The survey produced at the end of the welfare adviser's first 4 months in post was accepted by the Council as the basis for the future functioning of the service.

Grafting a social work agency that offered support to an individual nurse involved in the disciplinary process of the Council on to its established structure was not an easy task. Extreme caution was necessary to ensure that the service was established on a firm legal base. It is interesting to note that, according to the orginal terms of reference in 1972, the service through its professional staff could only become involved in a case once the Disciplinary Committee had made a decision. During the ensuing years the role of the service was subjected to continuous review and evaluation as a result of which its remit has now been extended to cover any nurse (qualifed or learner) involved in, or at risk of becoming involved in, the Council's disciplinary function.

The model on which the service is based is the statutory Probation and After-Care Service. There are many similarities between the two in that probation officers are social workers operating in a court setting and the clients of the Nurses Welfare Service, many of whom have already been convicted in court, are identified by their connection with the disciplinary function of the Council. Experience in statutory probation has always been regarded as the most appropriate for the welfare adviser's role, and all the professional qualified social workers who have been employed in the service to the present (1980) have had probation experience.

The relationship between the Council and the service is one of sensitivity, delicacy and mutual trust. Some people find it difficult to understand how a statutory body with responsibility for taking disciplinary action against individual nurses can at one and the same time offer the helping hand of a welfare service. Firstly, these two concepts are *complementary* rather than contradictory, provided you accept the basic premise that professional discipline is about the protection of the vulnerable public and not about punishment. Secondly, the help and support offered must be, and must be seen to be, separate from the body taking the disciplinary action. This is vital from the point of view of potential clients, as it must be abundantly clear to them that they can enter into relationships of trust with the welfare advisers in the certain knowledge that none of the information shared in the course of an interview will be passed on to anyone without their prior consent. To emphasise the separate nature of the service, a charitable trust was set up from the outset and is responsible for its funding and general administration. The trust is largely financed by voluntary donation, which causes certain problems in an age of high inflation. An added difficulty is that the work of the service is not immediately obvious to most people as a worthwhile cause to be supported. The existence of the trust, however, has given the service professional independence by making the staff accountable directly to the trustees rather than the Council. This is a key factor in the way that potential clients perceive the service, as it helps to underline its totally confidential nature. Having emphasised the need for separation from the Council, it should also be borne in mind that by definition the service must have a close working relationship with the statutory body, from which it derives its credibility, to a considerable extent its respectability, and its raison d'être. The last point is particularly crucial because of the element of suspicion that often lurks in people's minds about voluntary agencies.

The Nurses Welfare Service is, therefore, a social work agency, staffed by professional qualified social workers, which exists to provide casework help and support for any nurse (qualified or learner) involved in, or at risk of becoming involved in, the disciplinary function of the General Nursing Council. The fundamental premise on which the service is based is that of a voluntary contract between client and welfare adviser. Whatever the source of a referral the potential client must always indicate his or her consent before one of the welfare advisers may intervene in a case. A carefully worded introductory letter explaining the role of the service is sent to all potential clients, who are free to either accept or reject the offer.

Potential clients may come from one or more of the following sources—self-referral or referral from a social worker (especially probation officers), a nurse manager or the General Nursing Council for England and Wales. With regard to the latter, a procedure was established by which the initial notification of conviction from the police, or details of an allegation of professional misconduct from an employing authority or private individual, and each subsequent document are sent to the senior welfare adviser by the deputy registrar of the Council. On the basis of a potential client's need and the resources currently available, the senior welfare adviser then exercises his or her professional judgement in selecting those cases in which an offer of help is made. The timing of such an offer is vitally important and can vary according to the circumstances of each case. In some instances the need for intervention becomes more apparent at a later stage in the development of a case than in others; for example, when a statement or explanatory letter has been received from the nurse concerned.

The representation at a disciplinary hearing provided by a lawyer or staff organisation and the casework support provided by the Nurses Welfare Service differ. Both are relevant and in many instances the two roles complement each other. The representative is committed to obtaining the best possible outcome of the case for the client, whereas the welfare adviser is concerned with trying to help the client to face the reality of a situation, even though it may be very painful at the time. Case 12 will help to illustrate the point.

CASE 12

A 35-year-old SRN was reported to the Council by the police, as a result of a conviction in court for stealing ampoules of pethidine and phenobarbitone. The court had made her the subject of a probation order for two years. She had over a period of time been employed in various hospitals, and had been the subject of many reports to the Council, all concerning the misappropriation of drugs. The reports, however, had always been presented belatedly after she had been dismissed, thus moving the problem on rather than confronting it. This happened on twelve occasions in little more than a year and the belated reports upon which it was not possible to act revealed a steadily worsening situation. The circumstances reported always concerned a box of pethidine that supposedly had fallen out of the drug cupboard when it was opened.

At last a district nursing officer was faced with a situation in which the nurse misappropriated and used drugs, the consequence of which was that she was unfit for duty. She quickly involved the police, channelled the nurse to appropriate medical help, and accompanied her to the subsequent court hearing. It emerged that the nurse had been suffering from depression after a gynaecological operation, and this state had been exacerbated by problems in her relationship with her parents. Whilst in a state of depression she had obtained the drugs and administered some of them to herself by injection. This led to her being found unconscious on the ward.

Shortly after the court hearing one of the welfare advisers became involved in the case, initially by liaising with the probation officer. During the intervening period before the Disciplinary Committee hearing a considerable amount of work was done with the nurse in trying to get her to face up to the reality of her serious drug addiction problem. She was helped to develop sufficient insight to attend the

Disciplinary Committee hearing, knowing that, because of her addiction problem, for her to remain on the Register would not be in her own best interest nor that of her patients.

She impressed the Committee members as a thoughtful, intelligent woman. She explained to them that she was undergoing treatment for her drug problem and had obtained employment outside nursing for the time being as she felt this would assist in her rehabilitation. She also indicated that she would at some later date like to resume nursing if possible. The decision of the Committee was to remove her name from the Register, after which she continued to have the support of the service.

The service, in 1980, was staffed by three professionally qualified social workers, with a collective experience of more than 20 years, and a secretary who fulfils the role of an anchor person in the office. Having England and Wales as a catchment area is a daunting prospect and the nature of the work is such that the professional staff are required to travel extensively, visiting clients in their own homes. In general it is possible to achieve far more by a home visit rather than by an interview at the office, both from the client's and the welfare adviser's point of view. The former normally feels more relaxed and able to talk freely in in the security and familiarity of his or her own home. A home visit is also a demonstration of a caring attitude on the part of the welfare adviser for the client, especially when the visit involves a long journey from the office base. Clients often feel guilty at the prospect of a welfare adviser embarking on a very long trip at their behest, and are reassured that nurses with similar problems do in fact exist some of whom are living in their own locality. To make travel as cost effective as possible it is planned in such a way as to take in visits to as many clients as possible on a particular trip.

The experience of the service over the past 7 years demonstrates that working with a client group of fellow professionals in a pioneering field of social work demands very special skills. A number of nurses have difficulty accepting the need for help either because of a lack of insight into a particular problem (e.g., alcoholism—a problem which showed a dramatic increase during the 1970s) or because such an acceptance is perceived as a sign of weakness or an admission of defeat. There is the added difficulty for all of us in the caring professions that to be in receipt of any form of care is a reversal of roles.

Home visiting has its lighter moments: the senior welfare adviser went to visit a new client some years ago to be greeted on the doorstep with a request to unblock her drains which had seized up. Being only too familiar with such catastrophes in his own domestic life he set to work on the drains and achieved a reasonable measure of success. It seemed that the man from the welfare in his best city suit had to perform some tangible mundane task before the client was willing to trust him with her personal problems. The drain incident helped to establish rapport and the client was helped through a difficult time involving removal from the Register and working towards the eventual goal of restoration which occurred some 18 months later.

In general terms the welfare advisers work directly with those clients who are not receiving any support from any other social work agency. In cases where a social worker colleague is already involved the service performs a liaising function, advising about the professional implications of a conviction. Increasingly the service is being used in a consultative capacity by social work and nurse colleagues. As more nurse managers have become aware of its existence there has been a significant increase in the number of early referrals, enabling the service to intervene at a point when help is most needed, rather than trying to pick up the pieces afterwards.

The main focus of the service is on short-term crisis intervention work during the period that clients are actually going through the Council's disciplinary procedures. As the service has become involved earlier in the development of cases clients are helped to understand the purpose of the Council's investigation and how it operates. Anxiety is allayed and what seems to most nurses the very complicated machinery which surrounds the disciplinary process is simplified. The welfare advisers never cease to be amazed at the sort of fantasies some nurses have about the powers of the Council. The first question put to one of them recently by a very experienced SRN who had been given an official police caution after helping herself to pethidine to alleviate the severe pain she was experiencing from burns was: Will the GNC send me to prison?

In addition to the short-term work undertaken, each welfare adviser carries a nucleus of long-term cases. For the most part this is made up of nurses whose names have been removed from the Register or Roll and who have opted to have continuing contact with the service in the hope of eventual restoration. This part of the work can at times be most difficult and frustrating, yet it is often the most rewarding. Convincing a client of the futility of applying for restoration before the ink has dried on the removal letter is a common experience for all welfare advisers. By making a premature application for restoration the client risks further rejection by his of her profession which can be very damaging to someone in an already fragile state. There are occasions, however, when in the professional judgement of the welfare adviser working with the client, an application for restoration with little or no chance of success should be allowed to proceed. Case 13 provides a good example.

CASE 13

An SRN was removed from the Register following a conviction for being jointly involved with her husband in using an instrument to procure an abortion that resulted in the death of the expectant mother. The client's husband had been sent to prison, and she received a suspended prison sentence. At the original hearing before the Disciplinary Committee she claimed that she had been coerced by her husband. While the Committee were not convinced at the time it was noticeable that as soon as he was discharged from prison he applied on her behalf for her name to be restored to the Register. She concurred with his initiative and proceeded with the application which was unsuccessful. The experience of being further rejected by her own profession acted as a stimulus for her to aim at a specific objective, that is, the need to prove to the Committee that she was an independent person in her own right, free from her husband's influence in her professional life. About a year later she made a second application supported by two excellent references from two senior nursing officers with whom she had been working as a nursing auxiliary, and who had full knowledge of the facts. Having convinced themselves by careful questioning that, in addition to the kindness, skill and care that referees spoke of, she had matured professionally and developed insight, the Committee members agreed to restore her name to the Register.

While helping clients through the disciplinary process of the Council, the service also assists the two Committees (responsible for professional discipline) in their decisions by providing social background reports. The purpose of preparing such reports is to enable the Committees to see the incident involving professional misconduct in its context from the point of the nurse's personal and professional life. Frequently, a social background report reveals a catalogue of disaster of such magnitude that one is left wondering how the particular nurse in question managed to keep going for so long. The reports also help to provide a backcloth against which a moment's aberration is seen in the context of perhaps 20 years' unblemished, committed, professional service.

The preparation and presentation of social background reports is the part of the welfare adviser's role most akin to that of the probation officer. As former probation officers now working in the Nurses Welfare Service, all welfare advisers cherish the commission to 'advise, assist and befriend' their clients. Yet at the same time they are fully aware of their additional responsibilities towards the protection of the vulnerable public. In preparing a social background report the welfare adviser attempts to make a comprehensive, objective, honest appraisal of the client and his or her circumstances. Nowhere is the precarious tightrope of the welfare adviser more evident than in this situation.

Before presentation to the Disciplinary Committee the social background report is shown to the client who can either agree to its presentation or refuse to have it presented. If the client agrees he or she is given the opportunity by the chairman to raise any points in it during the proceedings. The majority of clients of the service are only too pleased to have such reports presented so that the Committee are made aware of their total situation. Further, a significant number of the nurses who come before the Disciplinary Committee do not have any form of representation as they do not belong to a staff organisation, and cannot afford to employ a solicitor privately. The number of social background reports presented to the Disciplinary Committee has been steadily growing. For example, in 1977 there were 37 reports; in 1978, the number increased to 47, or by 27 per cent; and by the start of 1980, social background reports showed an increase of 89 per cent over three years.

The term *welfare* is by its very nature somewhat nebulous. In this particular context it tends to conjure up the picture of social workers dispensing tea and sympathy to nurses who have been struck off the Register. The Nurses Welfare Service sets out to achieve more than this. It provides a casework/counselling service for its nurse clients, enabling them initially to identify the underlying factors which have led to their involvement in the Council's disciplinary process. Secondly, it assists them to formulate realistic plans about working through the problem areas. Having established a casework contract with the client involving honesty and mutual trust, it is then possible for the welfare adviser to use the Disciplinary Committee's decision as part of a plan to achieve a certain objective. For example, a nurse who has been removed from the Register because of a drink problem is told by the chairman that this is not necessarily the end of his or her career and that it is possible eventually to apply for restoration. Such a decision can provide the client and welfare adviser with the ideal opportunity to sit down together and discuss how best they can tackle the problem together, with restoration as the ultimate goal.

Establishing rapport with the client can be a difficult, painstaking exercise in which the welfare adviser frequently absorbs a lot of pent-up aggression, and even risks physical attack. On one occasion a senior welfare adviser was given the chance to demonstrate his prowess as a slip-fielder when an angry client hurled her badge across the room at him. The client, dismissed from her nursing post and subjected to considerable publicity in the local press as a result of her conviction in court, faced the prospect of the breakup of her marriage. The letter from the Council inviting her statement or explanation was the final straw so far as she was concerned. Her initial reaction was to say that she did not want any more to do with nursing and used the senior welfare adviser (whom she saw as the human face of the General Nursing Council for England and Wales) as the butt of her aggression. She needed many hours to talk through her feelings before she could admit that she cared very deeply about her professional qualification and did not want to lose it. She came to the Disciplinary Committee hearing supported by her husband and former senior nursing officer. The Committee decided to postpone judgement for a period of one year. The case was satisfactorily completed, and the client is working again as a staff nurse.

The location of the service is an important component in the way that potential clients perceive its role. Initially, the welfare advisers operated from the General Nursing Council offices, where the service remained for the first four years of its existence. Subsequently, however, the view has been that separate premises are more satisfactory and help to ensure that the clients see the service as being completely separate from, while associated with, the Council.

In addition to the casework undertaken with clients in need, the service shares with certain Council staff a responsibility to make the nursing profession more aware of the concept of professional discipline and the support services available to nurses subject to the Council's disciplinary process. This responsibility is fulfilled by all three welfare advisers speaking at study days and seminars for nursing personnel at every level all over Great Britain.

The creation and development of the Nurses Welfare Service has effected something of a revolution in the professional disciplinary processes operated by the Council. Many members now say that they would find it impossible to serve on the Disciplinary Committee if the service did not exist. Presently, removal from the Register or Roll of Nurses can be, and often is, a contribution—maybe the first step—towards the rehabilitation of a nurse, because realistic and understanding support is available on a continuing basis. The many nurses who have received support at difficult times in their lives, and have become suitably rehabilitated, are excellent evidence to the need for and the achievements of the Nurses Welfare Service.

8

Lessons, Problems and Failures

If reasonable standards of nursing care are to be available to the public, the nursing profession must consider continuously its methods and skills and evaluate its performance of those skills. When a wilful breakdown of performance occurs, the profession through its disciplinary process must deal with the offence and the offender to protect the offended. Thus far, we have examined the structure, composition and proceedings—general and specific—of the disciplinary process; let me now ask:

What lessons emerge from observation of the professional disciplinary process about the members of the nursing profession?

What lessons emerge from observation of the professional disciplinary process about nurse managers?

What lessons emerge from observation of the professional disciplinary process about employing authorities?

What points arise about the effectiveness of staff organisations in representing their members?

What points arise about the General Nursing Council for England and Wales and its procedures?

What questions arise about the range of decisions available to the relevant Committees of the Council?

What lessons emerge from observation of the professional disciplinary process about the members of the nursing profession?

I deliberately take this question first, because the answers to it are so disturbing and wide ranging, and because it forms the context within which the other questions must be asked and answered. Whenever I attempt to answer this question and the subsequent questions at seminars or conferences I find myself saying with almost monotonous regularity We fail. Following those words, I expound the ways in which

71

we (that is the qualified nurse members of the profession in the United Kingdom) fail, if the evidence of the professional disciplinary work of the statutory bodies is to be believed.

Often I am taken to task by a member of my audience (sadly it is usually a nurse teacher) for suggesting that such 'failure' is general when my evidence, though based on a large number of cases, is the result of the culpable actions of a small percentage of the working nurse population. While I am always willing to accept the latter point, I find it necessary in reply to express the conviction that not all those nurses who are, for example, found to be misappropriating drugs or are failing to provide appropriate care to their patients, are reported to the Council and become the subject of disciplinary proceedings. My conclusions are open to challenge, but I am yet to be convinced that they are not reasonable conclusions, and I have to state them because very often they are about the settings in which we seek to educate nurses.

What are my conclusions? Basically these:

i. *That we often fail to educate nurses to understand what it means to be members of a profession.* So often those who have qualified as nurses see their role only in terms of a job with its rewards, rather than as professional employment with its large responsibilities. (Case 4 in Chapter 2 illustrates what I mean, as do several of the case studies in Appendix A.)

ii. *That we often fail to educate nurses to understand what professional responsibility means.* I appreciate that in saying this I am iterating some material from Chapter 1, but it seems important to restate my conviction that *all* qualified nurses have:

a. a responsibility for their own standards of patient care, and for developing their skills and perceptions
b. a responsibility to participate in the teaching of others
c. a responsibility for the settings in which patients are cared for
d. a responsibility for their colleagues

All too often the picture that seems to emerge from the professional disciplinary work of the General Nursing Council for England and Wales is of a 'profession', many of whose members think that it is none of their business what their colleagues are doing, that it is only for the nurse managers to trouble themselves about the settings in which patients are cared for, that if they wanted to teach they would have become tutors or clinical teachers, and that they had achieved the ultimate when they obtained their nurse qualification and have no need of further development. Thankfully there are many known to you and me who do not match this sad and possibly offensive statement, but I ask you to regard it as much more than a caricature.

What lessons emerge from observation of the professional disciplinary process about nurse managers?

To offer my answer to this question I must refer you back briefly to the preceding section, for I maintain that all the responsibilities that are those of any qualified nurses must be those of nurse managers also. But simply because they are managers they have additional responsibilities. Again I repeat some points made in Chapter 1, but I also develop them for the purposes of this chapter.

First, they have the additional responsibility of maintaining and sustaining a setting which is dynamic, so that nurses (not just those in training) may grow and improve, and thus contribute to the growth and improvement of others. This is not only (indeed not even mainly) about equipment, but much more about attitudes.

Second, they have a responsibility to the public to ensure that those they employ as registered or enrolled nurses are such, and to accept that in respect of engaging nurses for employment you cannot and must not assume anything. After all, it would be possible for a member of the public to allege to the Council that a nurse manager was guilty of professional misconduct for failing to make all appropriate checks, as a result of which an unqualified person was taken into employment for which a registered or enrolled nurse was required. This is no mere hypothesis.

The fact that any person is able to talk himself or herself into employment for which he or she is not qualified amazes me, but it happens many times each year in spite of the facilities provided for checking claimed qualifications. If that amazes me, then I have to say that I am staggered at the fact that, on occasions, persons whose names have been removed from the Register or Roll of Nurses following criminal convictions, and as a result of a Disciplinary Committee public hearing attended by a senior nurse manager from the authority concerned, and whose names as 'removed' persons have been widely circulated by the Council, step straight into advertised nursing posts, and sometimes in the very locality where they committed the offences that led to conviction and removal!

Third, nurse managers have a responsibility for the settings in which patients are cared for which is far greater than the same responsibility of nurses at large, simply because they are employed in positions which enable them to make appropriate representations. They bear this responsibility not only that the patients may receive safe and competent nursing care but that the nurses working in those settings are not rendered vulnerable by excessive pressure.

Last, if we are to have even just reasonable standards of patient care and if we are to deserve that word *profession*, nurse managers have a responsibility to avoid 'sweeping things under the carpet', or, put another way, to avoid abrogating their responsibility.

So to return to my question, 'What lessons emerge . . . about nurse managers? I suggest:

i. That some nurse managers allow themselves to be party to a system which fails to prepare enrolled nurses for the responsibilities they are to bear, or which uses them in ways for which their training was neither designed or intended to prepare them.

I cannot hide the concern I feel at the fact that we go on taking into nurse training two categories of people of two quite different levels of academic attainment and

a. submit them to training programmes of different duration, content and levels of demand

b. test them by different examinations for which the depth and range of knowledge are markedly different

c. then send them out into a world where they will be used as interchangeable people.

Because this happens so much it comes as no surprise to me that a significant number of enrolled nurses find themselves involved in the Council's disciplinary process simply because they have found themselves 'in charge' in situations for which their training had not prepared them (indeed was not intended to prepare them), and in which they could reasonably have expected not to have to bear such responsibility. Is it not part of the nurse manager's responsibility to resist this disturbing trend?

ii. That some members of the profession (even some in quite senior positions) seem all too willing to abrogate their personal professional responsibilities to others, sometimes seeking short-term solutions with no thought for the long-term consequences.

I recognise that there is a danger in what I have just written. Some may read it as an attack on nurse managers, but it is not intended as such. Rather it is an attempt to remind them of a key responsibility and to encourage them to face up to it. Many do just that, and I respect them for the courage and integrity that they show, often in extremely difficult situations, where the demands far exceed the capacity of limited financial resources to provide. There are still those, however, who do not seem to fight to ensure that authority members have professional nursing advice when dealing with matters concerning professional nurses. Moreover, there are still those who take the view that unless a nurse has been the subject of dismissal which has not been successfully challenged, no matter how professionally reprehensible the offence, no report will be made to the General Nursing Council. This is to be deplored, as also is the practice of allowing a quiet resignation in exchange for a guarantee of no report and therefore no disciplinary action (see case 7 in Chapter 2 for an example of the consequences). It was in response to both such situations that the General Nursing Council for England and Wales issued its circular 77/13 in July 1977. It reads:

BASIC EXPLANATION OF THE COUNCIL'S DISCIPLINARY RESPONSIBILITIES

1. The Council's Senior Officers currently spend a significant amount of time in answering questions which illustrate the confusion that exists for many people (including nurse managers) between those issues which are matters for decision by employing authorities, and those which require the collective professional judgement of the relevant Committees of this Council. This confusion becomes still more evident in certain statements made before the Disciplinary Committee. For this reason the members of the Disciplinary and Investigating Committees consider it advisable to issue this Circular.
2. Rule 42 of the Nurses Rules, Approval Instrument 1969 (Statutory Instrument 1969 No. 1675) reads:

INVESTIGATING COMMITTEE

42. (1) When it is brought to the notice of the Council that a registered nurse has been convicted of a crime, or where [he or] she is alleged to have been guilty of any misconduct, during the period in which [his or] her name is in the register . . . the Registrar, after making such further inquiries relative thereto as [he or] she thinks necessary, shall invite the respondent to furnish any written statement or explanation which [he or] she may desire to offer and shall lay the matter before the Investigating Committee.
(2) The Investigating Committee shall consider the matter and may at any stage of the case take the advice of the solicitor, and may instruct him [or her] to obtain proofs of evidence in support of the allegations against the respondent, and may, in such cases as they think fit, decline to proceed with the matter.
(3) Where the Investigating Committee decide that the case is one in which the nurse shall be cited to appear before the Committee they shall refer the case to the Committee and may direct the solicitor to take all necessary steps for verifying the evidence to be submitted to the Committee and for obtaining the necessary documents and the attendance of witnesses.

There are Rules to similar effect for enrolled nurses, student and pupil nurses, candidates for examination/assessment, and applicants for registration/enrolment. (Subsequent Rules in each set give further specific details as to the process to be followed in cases that begin within the context of the Rules referred to above.)

3. It should be noted that the Rules read as they do, and do not make the submission of a report about a nurse to this Council dependent on a dismissal which is not successfully challenged. To make it so dependent would mean (for example) that nurse managers abrogated their personal professional responsibilities, since in effect lay members of Area Health Authorities or Industrial Tribunals would, in making a decision about employment, be making a further professional decision which is not theirs to make.

4. The Rules referred to place upon the Council an unequivocal responsibility:

(a) to investigate those matters brought to its attention (whatever the source);

(b) to decide, in those cases which are not the result of findings of guilt in court, whether the allegations are proved beyond reasonable doubt;

(c) to decide, in all proven cases, if the facts constitute professional misconduct; and

(d) to decide, in all cases considered professional misconduct, what is the appropriate collective professional judgement.

5. This collective professional judgement is a requirement of the law aimed at determining the appropriateness of a person to continue to hold the right to practise as a registered or enrolled nurse (or in the case of a student or pupil nurse to make a decision concerning their eventual admission to the Register or Roll). As such it must be exercised without reference to the employer's decision as to whether a person should or should not continue in his or her employment, although that person's previous professional performance will clearly be taken into account. In the majority of cases this will have a mitigating effect.

6. Conduct that an employing authority decide justifies dismissal will not necessarily be deemed professional misconduct, and vice versa. There are two quite separate decisions to be made by two different groups of people, both of whom have responsibilities under different sections of the law of this country.

7. It is often the case (in respect of registered or enrolled nurses) that an incident that leads to consideration of a nurse's position as an employee also necessitates consideration of his or her right to practise. The latter consideration cannot be dependent on, and should not be delayed by the former. It must be remembered that a professional nurse is subject to all the contraints of the criminal law, and is controlled and supported by Industrial Relations law as are other citizens. However, it must also be remembered that he or she is additionally subject to the requirements of nursing legislation, the purpose of which is the protection of the public. It is therefore incumbent on nurse managers to draw to the attention of the Council any matters that they consider to be of professional concern, irrespective of the decisions made concerning employment.

8. This clarification is issued for the guidance of nurse managers, and additional copies are provided for the information of regional, area and district personnel officers. Questions arising from this Circular should be addressed to the deputy registrar (Extension 51) or in his [or her] absence to the registrar (Extension 50). (A brief summary of the disciplinary process and philosophy is contained in an Appendix to this Circular.)

APPENDIX

1. The General Nursing Council for England and Wales is required by law to exercise a 'Professional Disciplinary' function.
The function is not punitive, but is intended:
   (a) to protect the vulnerable public;
   (b) to maintain professional standards; and wherever possible
   (c) to rehabilitate the nurses concerned.

2. This function is exercised through two of the Council's Committees. First, the Investigating Committee, which can decide:
   (a) that the matters reported are of no concern to the Council;
   (b) that the matters reported are of concern, but that some words of caution and counsel are sufficient;
   (c) that the matters reported necessitate a hearing before the Disciplinary Committee.

3. Second, the Disciplinary Committee which (if it considers misconduct to be proved) can:
   (a) administer a caution, but take no further action;
   (b) place the nurse concerned on Postponed Judgement (this is basically an opportunity for a person to prove herself or himself, with support, before a final decision is made);
   (c) remove the nurse's name from the Register or Roll of Nurses.

4. Cases originate from (a) findings of guilt in criminal courts, and (b) allegations from the work situation. In the first category the conviction has to be accepted, but in the second category (unless the nurse admits in advance) the allegations are unproven until found otherwise by the Disciplinary Committee as a result of their consideration of the evidence.

5. The Committee always endeavour to consider an offence in its context.

6. Whatever the decision of either Committee, the professional social workers who staff the Nurses Welfare Service can become involved in caring for the nurse, provided that their offer of help is voluntarily accepted.

iii. That nurse managers frequently fail to recognise the stress to which they submit their most reliable staff.

I hope that I have sufficiently illustrated what I mean through the cases numbered 5 (Chapter 2) and 11 (Chapter 6). It is a matter of great concern to me that the moral of those cases (and they are not unusual) is that you should not acquire a reputation for being very reliable. How sad it is that I should have had to arrive at that conclusion, but the evidence is there for all to see. Thankfully I also observe

the reverse of this phenomenon, and am pleased to know nurse managers who, through all their own difficulties really care for and about the
staff for whom, and to whom, they have a very special and well-fulfilled
responsibility.

What lessons emerge from observation of the professional disciplinary
process about employing authorities?

While I readily accept that there are many authorities, with varying
numbers of nurses in their employment, which do not deserve any or
all of my strictures, I must generalise, and assume that those who are
innocent in any or all respects will understand and re-examine their
policies and procedures. Are all employing authorities creating and
sustaining settings in which both their nurse employees and the senior
nurse managers (and all other health professionals) can perform their
duties and achieve the goals for which they were engaged in an atmosphere that does not render them professionally vulnerable?

Although there is some overlap between this and the preceding
section, it is inevitable and does not invalidate my arguments under
either heading. What are my points about employing authorities?

The most significant lesson I have learned (from the professional
disciplinary process) about employing authorities is that they sometimes expect the impossible, and thereby are often likely to do the most
harm to those whose professional commitment makes them strive to
achieve the impossible. (Case 6, Chapter 2, and case 11, Chapter 6
illustrate this point.) Nurse managers of different levels were involved
in both cases, but does that absolve members of health authorities from
any responsibility for the true facts? I say that it does not. In its Annual
Reports for 1978–79 and 1979–80 (reports which had to be submitted
to the Secretary of State for Social Services, and could not be released
until he had presented them to Parliament) the General Nursing
Council for England and Wales placed on record their concern that
such a significant number of cases appearing before the Disciplinary
Committee are a consequence of excessive and unacceptable pressures
in working situations.

The second lesson I drew from this work is that employing
authorities often seem to fail to realise that the nurse (or other statutor-
ily registered health professional) cannot be regarded in exactly the
same way as other employees. The nurses are responsible for their
actions not only to their employers but to the statutory body that
regulates their profession. While the authorities rightly have a role to
play in making decisions about a nurse as an employee, they may not
obstruct the professional registration body in its responsibility to make

a decision about an individual's appropriateness to continue to hold a statutory nursing qualification. Nor may they obstruct or influence their senior nurse managers who have the personal professional responsibility of deciding what matters should be reported to that body for a professional judgement. Case 14 touches on my meaning.

CASE 14

On a cold January night two nurses on a psychogeriatric ward decided on a course of action that led to their appearance before the Disciplinary Committee of the General Nursing Council for England and Wales some weeks later. One nurse was a part-time staff nurse (he also worked full-time with another authority), and the other a full-time enrolled nurse, and both were direct employees.

The circumstances were that a certain old lady was causing something of a disturbance in the early morning hours, and needed a lot of attention to quieten her. Looking on to the routine morning work that had to be done when the patients were woken, the two nurses agreed that this lady would be a disruptive influence and impede their progress, and together they resolved to seclude her in a room which was adjacent to the ward, though not a part of the ward. At about 5.00A.M. they placed the patient in the room, and were able to proceed with their routine morning work uninterrupted except for the death of a patient shortly before the change of shift.

No mention was made of the patient in question in the ward report, but as the night nurses were leaving they said to the staff nurse who had taken over (almost as a throwaway remark) that she was in the particular room. Because of the death which had just occurred, however, the staff nurse first turned her attention to contacting the relatives of the dead patient, and other associated duties. In consequence it was over half an hour after her arrival that she went to see the patient in the room indicated by the departing night staff. To her horror she found the patient clad in only an open backed nightdress, with no dressing gown, slippers or blankets, seated in a vinyl covered chair. The room was unlit and unheated, and the old lady was blue with cold. She could not have returned to the ward as there was no door handle on her side, and for the same reason she could not have put the light on. The staff nurse got the old lady back to her bed and took the necessary resuscitative measures, and then called her nursing officer to report what she had found.

As a consequence of her report, and the nurse manager's conviction that the situation had been as the staff nurse had described, the two nurses were dismissed from their employment. The circumstances were reported to the Council in a well-documented fashion by the divisional nursing officer, and the Council's procedures (investigation, statements from nurses involved, and the like) were followed. The Investigating Committee considered that the matters justified a hearing before the Disciplinary Committee, and the formal notices of the inquiry were sent out.

The hearing before the Disciplinary Committee took place on the scheduled date, but it was not possible to conclude it in the allocated time, so the particular group of Committee members had to decide when they could all meet to resume. However, between the incomplete hearing date and that fixed for the resumption an appeal by the enrolled nurse was heard by three lay members of the Area Health Authority. Largely on the grounds that there had been no previous offence meriting a final warning, the appeal was upheld and a final warning substituted. The appeal committee also decided that the same decision should apply to the registered nurse who had not appealed.

The district nursing officer then contacted the Council to ask that, as it was area policy only to allow the report to Council of offences that resulted in dismissal and as the dismissal of these nurses had now been rescinded, the Council stop its proceedings. She was told that the matter had come to the attention of the Council as the rules required, that it had been considered by the Investigating Committee to justify a hearing before the Disciplinary Committee, and that the adjourned hearing would resume on the planned date in accordance with the requirements of the Nurses Act and Rules approved by Parliament.

The district nursing officer would not have been put in that invidious position if the Authority members had been even just reasonably knowledgeable about nursing legislation, and the consequent professional obligations that such legislation places upon the nurse managers.

My third conclusion about employing authorities is—one that I levelled at some nurse managers—that of seeking short-term solutions to certain problems with no thought for the long-term consequences. This style of management (or should I call it expedient response?) often amounts to a failure to manage. I am disturbed by the degree to which committed conscientious nurse managers suffer when their decisions are overruled. Whenever this happens without sound reason another step is taken on the road to deteriorating standards.

What points arise about the effectiveness of staff organisations in representing their members?

The answer to this question must be prefaced by the comment that I find it surprising, after several years of rapid growth in the nursing membership of trades unions and professional organisations, that such a significant percentage of nurses appearing before the Disciplinary Committee of the General Nursing Council for England and Wales are members of none of these organisations and must, therefore, either attend without representation or sustain the cost of representation by a solicitor or barrister.

There is no need to attempt comparisons between the effectiveness of representation by lawyers and that of the officers of staff organisations, but as the latter are regularly involved they should be able to benefit from their accumulated experience. Although the following five points may appear to be generalising, they may be worth considering by the officials who attend to represent their members, and possibly improve the quality of representation.

i. Officers of organisations representing their nurse members often, surprisingly, fail to realise that a Disciplinary Committee composed totally or primarily of experienced nurses has a greater knowledge of the settings of nursing care, nursing hierarchies, of policies and procedures, than does an average appeal committee or Industrial Tribunal.

ii. On occasions I am surprised when a representative, speaking on behalf of a nurse appearing on a charge of misappropriation of drugs, stresses the small monetary value of the drugs and fails to note that the professional significance of the offence lies not in monetary value but in the nature of the drugs and the method of misappropriation. To say that the pethidine your client or member stole was worth only 25p hardly endears you to a committee of nurses. (If it is any comfort, some lawyers are guilty of the same error of judgement. I make the point because I expect better of organisations and officers who are in regular contact with the Council and its disciplinary prodecures.)

iii. It is not only surprising but shocking when a nurse's representative indicates to the Disciplinary Committee that he or she has already told the respondent that the offence is only a minor one and will result in a caution. This is exactly what a representative said to the Committee in case 5 (in Chapter 2). In so doing he was grossly underestimating the professional significance of the offence and failing to recognise the devious methods employed in committing it. By appearing to usurp the Committee's authority in this way the representative introduced an element of risk that the Committee would be more harsh than they would otherwise be to teach him (the representative) a lesson. (In the case quoted the Committee resisted that temptation—the nurse was placed on Postponed Judgement.) Unfortunately this is not an isolated example.

iv. Another point that continues to emerge with such consistency as to warrant comment is the practice that some representatives have of challenging the credibility of witnesses. They draw attention firmly and repeatedly to the fact that the complainants made their allegations only several weeks (or sometimes only days) later. This is a futile exercise when it is made to a committee who know hospitals, and know just how hard it is for first-year student nurse or a newly employed nursing auxiliary to bring their complaint into the open.

v. My final point is the most significant of the five because it is most often observed and because those representatives who make it demonstrate their failure to appreciate the Disciplinary Committee's role.

The Committee are often told by representatives that the respondent, convicted in a criminal court and dismissed from employment, has been punished enough, and that the Committee ought not to punish further. To say this, and in particular to make it the focal point of a submission on behalf of a respondent nurse, is unreasonable and sometimes even provocative. The Committee are there with a remit which requires them first and foremost to make what they believe is the necessary decision to protect the public and to maintain professional standards. The criminal courts exist to impose the punishment of society—the Disciplinary Committee has to decide whether a nurse whose guilt has been both established and considered professional misconduct might retain the right to practise. As I have said before, a nurse whose name is removed from the Register probably does feel punished on that day, perhaps for many days and weeks afterwards. Punishment, however, is not the Committee's role.

What points arise about the General Nursing Council for England and Wales and its procedures?

The procedures of the General Nursing Council for England and Wales in respect of its professional disciplinary responsibilities are, for the most part, defined in some detail in the Nurses Rules and Enrolled Nurses Rules. What is not explicitly stated in those rules has developed from and around them in a way that seems both to work and to be logical.

The procedures (detailed in Chapters 4 and 5) that have evolved are, in my personal view, working well. My deep involvement in the procedures may, at first glance, qualify me as the least satisfactory person to make any critical comment. Since 1974, I have explained the professional disciplinary procedures, method and available decisions to many thousand registered and enrolled nurses (at conferences, seminars, study days, management courses) received their response, answered their questions, encouraged many of the same people to come and see the Disciplinary Committee in action and talked with them about what they have seen and heard. I find that my opinion is the same as that of many other people. This collective opinion leads me to comment:

i. The reporting system by which cases begin in general works well. This general comment is made in the light of the points made about managers and employing authorities, and must obviously be qualified by those points. It is also intended to be comprehensive, in that it includes both cases reported by the police following the establishment of guilt in criminal courts and those which come to the Council by way of allegations made.

ii. The piece of the law which requires the appropriate officers of the Council to notify the nurse concerned that her or his conviction has been notified or an allegation made against her or him, and to invite an explanation or comment is regarded as of the greatest importance.

iii. The Council's practice of trying to set an offence or alleged incident in its work and career context, while not strictly required by the rules which set out the law, is widely held to be entirely correct.

iv. There is considerable anxiety expressed about the Investigating Committee. This anxiety has only come to the surface since 1978 as a consequence of a few well-publicised cases. Before that, the profession did not seem to notice that a small group of their colleagues bore this onerous burden on their behalf. The concern expressed is not about the role of the Investigating Committee—the majority seem to accept the need for a professional sieve—but rather that a small group of people (the Committee is eight, the quorum only three), meeting in private, have the power to prevent the Disciplinary Committee from ever considering certain cases, even if the rest of the nursing profession think they should be the subject of a hearing. Others, of course, are unlikely to have anywhere near as much information placed before them as has the Investigating Committee, but that does not necessarily rob their concern of its validity.

It would clearly be impractical to have a system wherein the Council (which includes the Disciplinary Committee) could overrule the Investigating Committee—this would be inconsistent with the legal delegation of function. Many do feel, however, that all is not well with this aspect of the present system, and I sympathise with their concern. At the Disciplinary Committee stage justice can be seen to be done, but not at the Investigating Committee stage.

One suggestion made frequently is that the Investigating Committee, like the Disciplinary Committee, should meet in public, but that in deference to its rather different role (professional sieve) a system should be devised which allows for the probability that it will send forward only about 30 per cent of the cases put before it, and the ensurance that anonymity is preserved in the remaining cases. This could be achieved by the Committee, meeting in public, hearing a brief verbal submission on the nature of the charge that would be laid if the matters were referred to the Disciplinary Committee. The members could reject the case at that stage or ask for further supportive information (drawn from police reports, witnesses' statements, respondent's explanation or comments) without divulging the name of the nurse or the place of the incident. The Committee members would then discuss the matter and arrive at a conclusion.

There is much to be said for this suggestion. It could not be implemented at present as it would necessitate changes in the appropriate statutory instruments. It should, however, be borne in mind as a distinct possibility for the future.

v. The Disciplinary Committee meets in public and for that receives wide acclaim from within the nursing profession. Many remark how important they regard its work, and how valuable they believe it that the many lessons contained in the cases it hears can be noted and applied in other places to avoid similar occurrences and to improve standards. While the Committee is required by law to meet in public, it is notable that they have the power under a particular statutory rule to hear evidence in camera when they consider it in the interests of justice to do so. That this rule exists but is only rarely used seems to be appreciated.

vi. The final point does not exactly match the question, and yet it needs to be made when considering the Council's procedures, as it is a matter of right and proper concern to many people. The concern (expressed to me by visitors to the Disciplinary Committee) is over the often long delay between an incident, and the appearance of the respondent before the Disciplinary Committee as a result of that incident. This matter is also of concern to me and to members of the General Nursing Council for England and Wales. It is hoped that the increase in the size of the Disciplinary Committee membership (to 16 from January, 1981) will resolve that part which is within their power to control.

Many delays, however, are outside the Council's power to control. It is not particularly difficult to progress a conviction case through the process described and get it to a Disciplinary Committee hearing in less than 2 months if it is deemed especially urgent. If the conviction, however, was the result of a crown court trial there may be a delay of possibly as long as $1\frac{1}{2}$ or 2 years between the incident and the court appearance. It is a great concern to many (and one I share) that a person may be charged with an offence which if proven would obviously be professionally serious, may be suspended on full salary for many months awaiting crown court trial, and may take up other nursing employment (e.g., through a nursing agency) in the meantime. As with point *iv*, this is a matter to which careful attention must be given, as delays before crown court hearings seem unlikely to shorten in the near future.

What questions arise about the range of decisions available to the relevant committees of the Council?

To assist the reader to arrive at an opinion on the points I now make, I will recap the available decisions and then comment.

1. *Registered and enrolled nurses*
(*a*) Criminal conviction cases
  The Investigating Committee, after considering all facts of the matter before them, arrive at:

DECISION. Of no concern to the nursing profession, and therefore there is no case to answer.

DECISION. Of concern (and therefore professional misconduct) but only such that a letter of caution and counsel will suffice.

DECISION. Of sufficient concern to justify a hearing before the Disciplinary Committee.
COMMENT. I believe this to be an entirely appropriate set of decisions. The only anxieties heard expressed relate to the procedures, and not to the available decisions.

  The Disciplinary Committee have first to decide whether they consider the particular guilt to be professional misconduct and if they do then they must arrive at:

DECISION. To administer a caution but take no further action.
COMMENT. This is obviously quite appropriate in those cases where the incident was relatively minor, where the nurse clearly understands the significance of his or her actions, is as near certain as can be not to repeat them, and on all the evidence is a competent and caring nurse and a safe practitioner.

DECISION. To postpone judgement for a stated time, thus leaving the nurse with the right to practise and the knowledge that at the end of a stated period the Disciplinary Committee will resume the hearing and will require (a) at least two references from people with knowledge of both the facts and the nurse's conduct during the intervening period and (b) other medical/psychiatric/social background reports as appropriate. It is made clear that the Disciplinary Committee have the same full range of options (including removal) open to them for the resumed hearing.

COMMENT. The empirical evidence proves this to be an effective decision for the large number of cases in which the Committee feel unable to close the matter with words of caution but feel removal from the Register or Roll to be too harsh. Statistics (see Appendix C) show that a majority of those placed on Postponed Judgement receive a caution at the resumed hearing because they have used the interim opportunity to prove themselves worthy of the Committee's trust. More significant, most respondents who come back to resumed hearings have apparently benefitted and developed insight as a result of their experience, and often have re-established themselves in employment and are performing to a high standard. For the few who do not use the opportunity presented the option to remove from the Register or Roll at the end of the period remains. The statistics show that it is used where appropriate. I believe that the Committee's postponement of judgement (as the criminal court's deferred sentence) to assess the respondent's progress is extremely valuable.

DECISION. To remove a respondent's name from the Register or Roll of Nurses, thus preventing him or her from practising in a professional nursing capacity.

COMMENT. It seems clear that any committee charged with the onerous responsibility of protecting the public must have this decision available to them. The acid test lies in whether it is used to achieve that objective, and not to punish the individuals involved. I believe it is properly used. In support of that is the considerable number of Removed nurses who are now restored, and whose rehabilitation seems to have begun from the date of their removal.

(b) Allegation cases

In allegation cases the Investigating Committee can only decide, on the basis of the information put before them (which will often include a letter of admission) whether if capable of proof the matters alleged are likely to be regarded as professional misconduct.

In the same type of case the Disciplinary Committee must first establish whether in their collective view, the allegations (unless already admitted) are proved beyond reasonable doubt. If they do so decide they must then follow the procedures and use the range of decisions already described for the conviction case.

GENERAL COMMENTS. While I consider each decision to have its place and maintain that each is used appropriately, I am only too aware (as are the Committee members, and I believe, many nurses who have come to observe the Disciplinary Committee in action) that for many nurses who are the subject of reports to the Council that lead to disciplinary hearings no decision is exactly right.

Consider the nurses who are guilty of offences that were committed in such circumstances that they must be regarded as culpable, but for whom those offences are the result of illness rather than wilful recklessness or villainy. Think also of those (who I cannot help at present) who clearly are not safe practitioners because they are temporarily ill, and who may well put their own professional life at risk by doing something wrong.

There are those who believe that the present range of decisions is too large. I believe that it needs to be larger still so as to deal with the problems referred to—but that is a question for the future.

2. *Student or pupil nurses*
(*a*) Training not discontinued in consequence of an offence
The situation is basically a simple one. The director of the school where the student or pupil nurse is being educated has (presumably) deliberately chosen to retain the person in the training programme. The Investigating Committee, as a result of their consideration of all the facts, must arrive at:

DECISION. Whether to accept that student or pupil's entry to a Council examination (success in which is an essential step in the route to the Register or Roll of Nurses).

If the Investigating Committee do not accept the entry the student or pupil's application must be considered by the Disciplinary Committee at a personal hearing. That Committee can reach:

DECISION. To accept or reject the application. If they reject it the person concerned can apply again at a later date and again have a personal hearing.
COMMENT. In general this aspect of the system works well. It is rare for the committees to have to use their power to reject an examination entry from a person whom the school director has supported, but I believe it to be a good thing that the law allows this where desirable.

(*b*) Training discontinued in consequence of an offence
Until 1980, the two committees had no power to prevent a discontinued learner from resuming training provided that the person was able to find a school of nursing to accept him or her for that purpose.

They now have that power (as they now also have power to ban a learner whose training has not been discontinued from remaining in that training).

If they choose not to exercise that power, and if the learner obtains a place in a school, it is the task of the Investigating Committee to arrive at:

DECISION. Whether the residue of training should be extended by virtue of the offence that made the consideration necessary. They can, if they wish, require the person to recommence the training from the beginning.

The Disciplinary Committee only enter into the case if the Investigating Committee have banned a resumption of training or have extended the training period because of the offence, and the learner is aggrieved at this decision and requests a personal hearing. This Committee also has no control over whether the person can obtain a training school place. Bearing in mind the nature of the offence they must simply reach:

DECISION. What training the learner must undergo if able to obtain a place. They have the power to invalidate all previous incomplete training.

COMMENT. This aspect of nursing law has been deemed unsatisfactory for a long time. By amendment of the statutory rules, a change has been made which would allow the committees to bar a student or pupil nurse who had committed a serious offence from resuming training until they decided in response to an application that it was reasonable. The rule amendments which allow for a ban on the resumption or continuation of training are entirely logical, since they introduce for the student/pupil category a situation that would be similar to the removal/restoration position for registered and enrolled nurses.

(c) Committing an offence between taking a Council examination and applying for admission to the Register or Roll

Again the position is relatively simple. When the learner commits an offence after completing the statutory training and passing the required examinations and then applies for admission to the Register or Roll, then:

DECISION. The Investigating Committee must either accept the application or refer it for a personal hearing before the Disciplinary Committee, which can either accept or reject the application.

If the Disciplinary Committee take the latter view it is the normal practice for them to indicate when they may be willing to consider another application (if made), and to set their criteria. In this way they pursue a course of action which is not unlike that for dealing with applications from Removed nurses for restoration to the Register or Roll.

COMMENT. The number of cases that fall into this category is small. I believe it to be only right that this means of controlling the route to the Register or Roll exists.

The professional disciplinary work of the bodies responsible for the regulation of the nursing profession must be studied openly and honestly. I believe that those who do this will find, possibly contrary to any preconceived ideas they might have had, that this is not about taking sides. All of the categories named (nurses, nurse managers, employers, staff organisations, statutory bodies) are on the same side in that they all should have the interests of the vulnerable public at heart, and all wish to provide a climate in which the best possible standards of care can be provided.

9

New Trends and Their Implications

Since the settings in which professional nurses perform their duties, exercise their judgement, and use their skills change constantly, it is inevitable that at least some of those changes are also reflected in the caseload of the committees responsible for the regulation of the profession through the professional disciplinary process. Certain changes are a consequence of new medical or surgical treatments or procedures that involve nurses in performing new treatments or employing new techniques. This can often mean that the opportunity for error or mistake is greater, as in consequence is the possibility of the nurse becoming the subject of allegations of professional misconduct arising from incompetence or carelessness.

When pressures increase because of innovations or new technology, they tend to be regarded as inevitable consequences of progress. The same cannot be said when the pressures in a setting for patient care change because while the workload remains static or increases the number of nursing staff available to perform that work declines. For those and a variety of other good reasons it seems logical that before looking at the future, we should look at some of the trends of the last few years and consider their implications.

The trend towards a larger number of cases warranting the consideration of the Investigating and Disciplinary Committees not only deserves but demands comment. This trend seems to be so firmly established as to be at one and the same time a present reality, and a near guarantee of a continued increase in numbers. When I make this point many people tend to presume the standards of members of the nursing profession (conduct, honesty, and the like), have deteriorated. It is an unfair and unreasonable generalisation. In fact, my personal view takes a quite different direction.

Clearly, as we have seen in earlier chapters, there has been an increase in cases requiring peer judgement. It is also clear that this prevails despite the cases of personal life and morality that used to be reported being either not reported now or regarded as of no concern. Paradoxically, I am encouraged by the increased reporting of certain types of case to the General Council for England and Wales. These cases coming more into the open direct the attention of the committee members to the fulfilment of their role as protectors of the public.

Why has there been simultaneous reduction in certain types of case and an increase in other types, the total effect of which has been to provide the relevant committees with more cases over-all, and to increase the complexity of the work to a situation where those committees are stretched to their limits?

First, why are there fewer cases that are concerned with personal morality? With certain quite appropriate exceptions, the attitudes of the nursing profession have changed in accordance with the pattern of attitude changes in society. To give birth to an illegitimate child now or to have an extramarital relationship does not attract the calumny that it would have 30 years ago (and possibly even more in the years between the wars). It is not surprising that such matters either are not reported to the Council or are largely disregarded if they are. Lest it be thought that any slackening of personal standards is inevitably reflected in all the decisions of those responsible for professional peer judgement in nursing, I hasten to add that evidence shows this is not the case where the matters have an obvious relevance to the profession. For example, although the general attitudes of society to drugs may be less responsible than we would wish, every disciplinary case that involves drugs is the subject of a deep and thorough analysis, and the police are required to report all convictions involving drugs no matter how small the quantity.

Next, let us consider a question which, at least in part, is the converse of the first. Why are there more disciplinary cases which require the consideration of the committees? I believe that there are several answers to this question. The most obvious is that there are more registered and enrolled nurses than there were in former years, and thus more who, if they are guilty of certain offences or named in certain types of allegation, will become the subject of a professional consideration to determine whether they may retain the right to practise as registered or enrolled nurses.

The remaining answers I can proffer are far less obvious and do not constitute an exclusive list. The reader may care to consider what answers he or she would give to the question. One answer I give is that I believe that the caseload is constantly growing because many members of the profession at large, nurse managers in particular, are becoming more aware of their total professional responsibilities and respond to that awareness in a most encouraging way. In less than a decade I observed a transition from a position wherein the work of the Investigating and Disciplinary Committees of the General Nursing Council for England and Wales was largely a 'taboo' subject to one wherein (sometimes on its own, but often within the larger context of professional responsibility or the law and the nurse or in parallel with industrial relations) it is much in demand for conferences, seminars, study days, management courses, and the like. As a result, many members are becoming informed and aware about a subject that formerly was largely a closed book.

While nurses retain their phantasies about the role of the Council in respect of professional discipline as being only punitive, it is not surprising when (out of what they believe to be loyalty) they look the other way when a colleague is misappropriating drugs from the ward stock and developing some drug dependence. It becomes a rather different matter when they learn that to bring their colleague's misdeeds—and her sickness—into the open can actually open the way to some specialist help being offered to assist in that colleague's rehabilitation. Many nurses have now come to appreciate that their responsibility to care for and about their patients and their responsibility to care for their colleagues are not incompatible and that professional integrity may sometimes necessitate reporting a colleague to their nurse managers.

If that is the case with members of the profession as a whole it is even more so with those who hold nurse management positions. There have been many such in the past who failed to report to the Council those things which they knew very well ought to be reported. Some may have taken this action out of kindness—they do not want the nurse who has either resigned or been dismissed to run the risk of losing his or her professional qualification. Some may have taken this action for the much less honourable reason that they did not wish to risk attracting unfavourable publicity for their hospital or community nursing service. Others, still, may have taken this action because they just did not know either how or even why their own profession was regulated. And some may have thought that they had solved a problem when in reality they had only moved it on.

There must have been many occasions in the past when nurse managers took a course of action which, while fulfilling their responsibilities to their patients at a particular time and in a particular place, neglected their other responsibilities to patients as a whole, to the profession as a whole, and to their possibly sick colleagues. The position has been changing in that nurse managers and nurse educators have been provided with considerable opportunities to become informed about this important aspect of nursing law.

Certainly the General Nursing Council for England and Wales has invested considerable resources in trying to close the serious information gap that has traditionally existed on this aspect of its responsibilities, and while that gap remains disturbingly large it is visibly shrinking. I observe with interest how the volume of telephone calls from nurse managers (wishing to discuss emerging problems of professional concern) rises after a conference or seminar in their part of the country, as does the submission of relevant complaints. In summary, I am convinced that the more the nursing profession's members are provided with, and accept, the opportunity to consider exactly what their professional responsibilities are, the less will things of concern be swept under the carpet. That can only be to the benefit of those who rely on the availability of a safe and competent nursing service!

A further answer for the increased number of cases that come to the attention of the General Nursing Council for England and Wales is that the public are more informed about the manner in which the nursing profession regulates itself, or at least more aware of how to obtain such information should the need arise. It is any citizen's right to bring a complaint about any nurse, and the Council must investigate such a complaint with the same thoroughness applied to a complaint from an employing authority or nurse manager. While the number of cases from this source is not large, it is becoming significant. In case 9 (Chapter 5) two visitors to a hospital ward brought allegations direct to the Council about the things which they had observed and considered reprehensible. Case A16 (Appendix A) provides another example for the reader's consideration. It would appear that neither case would have received the professional consideration they undoubtedly deserved had the complaints not been brought to the attention of the Council by members of the public. I can only welcome this recent development.

The next in my list of answers to the increased disciplinary caseload is one I find sad but necessary to state: that is, cases resulting from the unreasonable pressures of the working situation. The nurses involved, whose professional qualifications and subsequently means of earning a salary are in jeopardy, are very often overly kind, competent and caring people—the sort with a reputation for being extremely reliable. These are the people who, when their employers expect them to achieve the impossible, will actually try to do just that. Many accept that they could only do the best that they could in the available time, and regret that this inevitably meant that their patients did not receive the attention they deserved. Some, either directly or through their staff organisation, remonstrate with their managers. But some, out of sheer professional integrity and commitment, try to bridge the gap between the possible and the desirable—occasionally cracking in the effort and become the subject of complaints to the Council. It is to people like this—the most committed—that we often do the most harm. At least a report to the Council makes available the specialist assistance of the Nurses Welfare Service to assist rehabilitation. But, why do we drive nurses to the point where this becomes necessary? My concern at this disturbing trend and at no sign of it being reversed in the foreseeable future is profound.

The last answer for the growth of the disciplinary caseload is very different, and yet to some degree it has associations with or might even be the cause of some of the problems ventilated in the preceding paragraph. The core of this part is found in that increasingly used phrase 'the extended role of the nurse'.

My immediate position is that I hold no doctrinaire objections to the clinical role of the nurse being extended in certain circumstances. I do object, however, if an extended role is introduced without a full and detailed examination of its necessity and if its consequence is further increased burdens on an already overburdened nursing staff. By all means extend the clinical role of the registered nurse, but only if it has first been established that:

a. the reasons for that decision in a particular setting are completely valid

b. the increased workload can be accepted by the nursing staff concerned without unreasonably eroding the time they have available for their normal and necessary duties of patient care

c. the necessary enabling work of instruction and authorisation has been completed

d. all the doctors in the particular setting are in agreement about the particular task that is being delegated and the method by which it is to be performed

e. the registered nurses involved are willing to accept the delegated function and so indicate

The importance of items *a*, *b*, and *c* should be self-evident. I cannot overstress the importance of *d*, having now dealt with a number of cases which resulted from a nurse complying with the wishes of one doctor and incurring the wrath of another who has complained to the Council about the nurse's conduct. The point in *e* is also vital: No nurse should feel compelled to perform a duty outside the normal role to which he or she was appointed. While it may well be true that, should there be a mistake with resultant unfortunate consequences, the employing authority will meet the financial costs of any litigation, it will be the nurse alone who will have to face up to the professional consequences of his of her mistake should there be a complaint made which necessitates a professional disciplinary enquiry. The types of case that have presented under this general heading are threefold.

First, there are those referred to in my comment on *d*. Second, there are those which stem from the situation where, for example, a registered nurse having some extended authority in one hospital moves to another hospital where he or she does not—and the nurse not only proceeds as if he or she possessed the same authority but extends it further. (Case A10 provides an example of this phenomenon.) Third, there are registered nurses who get so carried away with the additional status or prestige they think accrues to them because they are doing 'doctor's work' that they neglect their basic nursing duties, and thus become the subject of complaints that require the judgement of their own professional peers.

I indicated earlier that I am encouraged by the increase in the number of cases. I am encouraged because the Council now finds itself dealing with the cases which really do require consideration. I refer especially to those cases which raise questions about the ways in which professional judgement and professional knowledge are or are not properly used—in short, *safe practice*. The trend that has brought such matters to the fore and which demands consideration of all its implications has to be good.

One other new trend, the potential implications of which are enormous, is not mentioned in my answers to the question Why more cases. . . ?, because the number of cases within this category is as yet very small. It needs to be examined, however, because it has been the subject of a large number of questions to the General Nursing Council for England and Wales in recent years, and finally the subject of much public comment, debate and discussion. It is the relationship between industrial action and professional misconduct.

From about 1976 onwards, in common with some other members of staff of the General Nursing Council for England and Wales, I frequently found myself faced with the task of answering enquiries of a new and interesting kind. By letter or telephone people were increasingly making contact to discuss or seek comments upon certain sets of circumstances which were usually presented in a rather hypothetical form. They were asked by district nursing officers (or other senior nurses with management responsibilities) or district administrators/ personnel officers, by senior hospital doctors, and by local officials of trade unions (e.g., branch chairmen, branch secretaries, stewards). All posed questions in general terms and usually described hypothetical circumstances towards: Is it professional misconduct to take industrial action (a) in any circumstances, and/or (b) in a particular set of circumstances (real or hypothetical)? The circumstances were then described.

From the first category the question tended to come as: Some members of the staff are suggesting that they might. . . . What advice if any should I give them about the possible effect of their actions on their professional status? From the second category it usually came as: The nursing staff are threatening to do this or refusing to do that, and my patients are being put at risk. Is that permissible? What are you going to do about it? From the third category the form of the question was more likely to be: These are the circumstances with which we are faced and in which we are having to work. The members are discussing possible action on this matter. Can I be told whether these possible measures will lead them into trouble with the General Nursing Council?'

To those who were calling or writing in their capacity as local branch officers of trade unions or professional organisations any answer would be prefaced by the recommendation that they also seek guidance from the head office of their organisation. In response to all categories the answer was that, in accordance with established practice,

the Council would look at any complaints made against nurses which arose from industrial action in their context

if it was alleged, however, that patients either suffered or were put at risk by such action (or inaction) the Council would have to investigate those allegations fully (just as they would any other allegations), and

if the allegations were proved it *may* put in jeopardy the professional qualifications of those registered or enrolled nursed involved.
In short, the advice was to think about and take a very careful measure of the circumstances and possible consequences before taking any decisions, and certainly before taking any action.

Answers of that kind, given to many different people over a period of about 3 years, were generally regarded as helpful contributions to the discusssions that were taking place in the various local settings. At no time was the answer given that what was being proposed or suggested was wrong—simply that all concerned should carefully weigh up all the circumstances, including the possible (no stronger than that!) ramifications for the professional careers of the registered and enrolled nurses who might be involved. Personally, I would certainly never have been tempted to state that industrial action by nurses (a) was necessarily wrong and (b) was necessarily professional misconduct, because there are rare circumstances in which some selective form of industrial action might be both a positive and a professional response on behalf of present and future patients. It would be pointless to give examples to illustrate such circumstances since professional nurses must always make judgements and decisions about the real situations in which they find themselves—not about someone else's hypothesis.

During 1979 the enquiries continued and were dealt with as described, but something new now happened. Several registered nurses became the subject of reports to the Council alleging professional misconduct arising out of industrial action which involved the withdrawal of labour and the reduction of service to and provision for patients. The relevant committees of the General Nursing Council for England and Wales dealt with those matters put before them on an individual basis, as did their counterparts in the Northern Ireland Council for Nurses and Midwives.

Whether stimulated by the events that led to the first such reports or by the general climate I cannot say, but during the first half of the 1979 the questions about industrial action and professional misconduct became more frequent. As a result of the nature and volume of those enquiries the General Nursing Council for England and Wales decided to release a statement on the subject in July, 1979. Together with an explanatory comment, it read:

'The General Nursing Council for England and Wales has decided to make a pronouncement on whether a nurse who limits or withdraws his or her services could face proceedings for professional misconduct.
'The Council is of the opinion that if a nurse puts the health, safety or welfare of his or her patients at risk by taking strike or other industrial action he or she would have a case to answer on the score of professional misconduct, just as he or she would if the health, safety or welfare of patients were put at risk by any other action on his or her part'.

RELATED COMMENT. This statement is made in the context of this Council's responsibilities in law which are concerned with entry to the profession, the maintenance of the Register and Roll of Nurses so that the public may know from whom safe and caring nursing service may be expected, and the regulation of the profession through the professional disciplinary process. All these responsibilities are concerned with the protection of the public. The Council takes this opportunity to remind all registered and enrolled nurses of their personal professional responsibilities, and emphasises its view that in choosing to become members of a caring profession nurses undertake responsibilities which need not necessarily be expected of others.

Much of the reaction to the statement was wondrous to behold, and the fact that the Council were simply stating in a widely distributed circular exactly what had been said by its officers to many group and individual enquirers over the preceding three years seemed to go unnoticed. A *Nursing Times* leader made a useful contribution to what became a very healthy debate:

> A nurse who strikes or takes some other form of industrial action which puts the patient at risk may be guilty of professional misconduct. A clear statement to this effect was agreed by the General Nursing Council for England and Wales last week, reminding us that 60 years on the statutory body's first duty remains the same: to protect the public.
> It is simply a statement of opinion and must not be taken to mean that every nurse who takes any form of industrial action will inevitably be struck off the Register or Roll. It does not make it illegal for a nurse to strike as it is for the police; nor does it bind the Council's own Investigating and Disciplinary Committees.
> So what is the point? First it takes us a little further down the path of defining professional responsibility—in choosing to be part of the nursing profession we opt for certain responsibilities which the lay public do not necessarily have.
> Second, the statement helps us to tackle the question raised so crucially in the Normansfield report—the conflict between the rights of patients and the rights of staff. The patient has the right not to be exposed to needless danger, while staff have a right to withdraw their labour in support of legitimate grievances. The GNC can provide no easy answers but at least we have now a basis for further debate.
> Third, the GNC has reminded us—implicitly—that while decisions to take industrial action are made collectively following national ballots of all members or at local meetings, the burden of professional misconduct falls on the individual. Unions or even branches of unions or groups of nurses cannot be referred to the Investigating Committee of the GNCs.
> Those who expected a hard and fast ruling from the Council after all the confusion and uncertainty of the Normansfield situation, will be disappointed. We have a statement which simply says that if a nurse puts the 'health, safety or welfare' of the patient at risk through industrial action, [he or] she would have a 'case to answer'.
> The onus falls on the Investigating Committee to show the patient had been put at risk and if so then the Disciplinary Committee would hear the case. But how do we define 'at risk?' If three out of six nurses in a ward strike, halving the normal cover, are the patients then at risk? If those same three nurses go off sick simultaneously and replacement staff cannot be found, should the ward sister demand that her ward be closed because the patients are at risk? It can only be a matter of opinion, but it must be professional opinion.
> And this is the crux. During the height of the industrial action last winter, there was talk of nurses and other NHS workers entering into a no-strike agreement in return for certain commitments from the

government on pay. Superficially this looks attractive, but professionally it would be dangerous. Strike action is the ultimate weapon which most nurses choose not to use in pursuit of claims on pay and conditions of service.

But what if, in [his or] her own professional judgement, a nurse feels [he or] she has no choice but to withdraw [his or] her labour in support of some issue concerning patient rights? The Disciplinary Committee could be faced with weighing up short-term risks against long-term ones.

The option to strike must be kept open but we must never put our own rights before those of our patients.

A *Nursing Mirror* leader approached the subject:

In a totally unambiguous statement this week, the General Nursing Council makes it quite clear that nurses who take strike action or any form of industrial action which puts at risk the health, safety or welfare of their patients could face a charge of professional misconduct. The GNC which has responsibilities for the maintenance of the Register and Roll, says any form of industrial action is legally indefensible.

Many nurses will believe that such a bold statement is a timely reminder following the troubled events of last winter and, in particular, at Normansfield Hospital where some nurses walked out on the mentally handicapped patients. The GNC adds: 'In choosing to become members of the caring profession, nurses undertake responsibilities which need not necessarily be expected of others'. We would like to support the stand being taken by the GNC. Service before self has always been one of the fine traditions of the nursing profession and nurses do have responsibilities to their patients which it would be foolish not to recognise.

However, nurses also have other responsibilities. Standards of nursing care are not advanced if nurses continue to leave the profession because of an unsatisfactory wage and if conditions in hospitals decline. Perhaps the means never justify the ends, but it is an unsavoury fact that conditions sometimes improve only after industrial action is taken, or the threat of it is made.

The Tories are keen to get no-strike guarantees in certain vital jobs in the public sector. The nursing profession as a whole, including the unions, should grasp this opportunity provided by the GNC of saying to Secretary of State Patrick Jenkin: 'We will surrender the strike weapon so long as you will give us in return certain guarantees over nurses' pay, possibly by index-linking it after the Clegg commission has made its proposals known'. We believe that such an opportunity should not be missed and the consequences of any repetition of last winter's anarchy too dreadful, if the profession and the Government do not take this chance

The *Nursing Mirror* continued to stimulate debate with a series of varied contributions over a period of several weeks.

Meantime there were many individual reactions from members of the nursing profession and officers of their various organisations. The statement was called ambiguous, unambiguous, preposterous, very welcome, of no value, an attempt to stop nurses from joining trade unions, disgraceful, timely, improper, a blow for freedom. Those which welcomed the statement for the clarification it had provided outnumbered the remainder. I suppose that one of the more frequently stated critical comments was that the Council were trying to rob nurses of their rights. However, the statement was not only about 'rights' but about 'responsibilities'. Reference to the dictionaries is useful in any consideration of this subject and these words. For example, *responsibility* is defined variously as : 'morally accountable for one's actions', 'liable to be called to account', and 'able to answer for one's conduct and obligations'. Interestingly, the word *Rights*, which in common use tends to have become a rather one-sided word, is defined as 'the standard of permitted and forbidden action within a certain sphere'. Using that definition it can fairly be said that the General Nursing Council's statement is about 'rights'.

Public debate continued over the latter part of 1979 and spilled over into 1980. The General Nursing Council for England and Wales demonstrated that all such cases were considered by the Investigating Committee in their context since of seven cases considered by them it was decided that there was no case to answer in five, while two were referred to the Disciplinary Committee for hearings, and those two nurses were subsequently the subject of postponed judgement decisions.

The points that emerged in the ensuing debate, and especially from the *Nursing Mirror* series of articles and the associated contributions to their correspondence columns, were many and varied. Differing points of view were rightly, sometimes forcefully, expressed. Clearly, some did not entirely understand either the statement and its implications or the background from which it was made. Eventually, as a result of and reaction to some of the criticisms or misunderstandings expressed, eight points required the same clarification publicly as had been given in many individual letters. They are that:

1. The statement is not about taking industrial action, not about the nurse's right to strike, not about trades union activity, not about management/staff relationships, allocation of resources or the many other issues raised by those who misunderstood or misinterpreted it. The statement is about the health, safety and welfare of patients, and the particular responsibility the qualified nurse holds to avoid placing patients at risk.

2. The statement mentioned 'strike or other industrial action' only because many people who had contacted the Council over the preceding months and years had been asking for clarification of the position where possible or threatened industrial action might result in some risk to patients.

3. There had apparently been some misunderstanding which had led some people to believe that actions which placed patients at risk would not be the subject of any action by the Council provided that they came within the general description of 'industrial action'. The statement set out to make it quite clear that those who held this view were wrong.

4. No nurse in the direct patient care situation who genuinely has the welfare of patients in mind and who demonstrates this in a carefully considered action need feel threatened by the statement; and no nurse manager who has struggled to obtain resources and use them responsibly, yet who is unable to provide the level of service he or she believes to be necessary, need feel at risk.

5. While the General Nursing Council for England and Wales must investigate all allegations made to it, each allegation is considered in its context, by committees drawn from a Council primarily composed of practising nurses who are thus well aware of the difficulties faced by nurses who have to meet an infinite number of demands from a finite amount of resources.

6. Because of points 1–5, the statement is not a threat to those who continue to provide the best possible care in often difficult circumstances; it is not a weapon to be used in a battle between individuals and organisations; and it is not a tool to be used by managers when they should be tackling a local issue of concern by the proper means of consultation and negotiation. It is, however, quite specifically about the individual nurse's professional responsibility to take a personal decision about any proposed or threatened industrial action, being sure to make the patients' health, safety and welfare his or her predominant consideration.

7. Rather than being seen as taking actions running counter to those of the trades unions and professional organisations who were seeking to effect improvements by drawing attention to the hazardous situations that exist, the General Nursing Council for England and Wales, through this statement and various others, were also drawing attention to those same hazards.

8. The Council was not, in this statement, breaking new ground, and applying new limits or constraints to qualified nurses who felt the need to take some action to improve their own lot or that of their patients or both. Various 'Codes of Practice' were prepared under the

terms of some previous industrial relations law but have remained in existence for guidance subsequent to the establishment of the Advisory Conciliation and Arbitration Service (ACAS). One such relevant code is:

> *Responsibilities—individual employee*
> Some employees have special obligations arising from membership of a profession and are liable to incur penalties if they disregard them. These may include, for example, those in regard to health, safety and welfare, over and above those which are shared by the community as a whole.
> A professional employee who belongs to a trades union should respect the obligations he [or she] has voluntarily taken on by joining the union. *But* he [or she] should not, when acting in his [or her] professional capacity, be called upon by his [or her] trades union to take action which would conflict with the standards of work or conduct laid down for his [or her] profession if that action could endanger:
> 1. public health or safety;
> 2. the health of an individual needing medical or other treatment;
> 3. the well-being of an individual needing care through the personal social services.

What, then, has happened since that few weeks of fairly intense debate following the release of the statement? While the enquiries of the sort that had steadily been increasing in volume over the months prior to the release of the statement did not cease altogether, they did decrease to very few, and are resolved by sending a copy of the circular that included the statement. Out of the debate, which in its early stages contained some acrimonious and illogical statements that are probably regretted and later moved on to quieter and more responsible exchanges, there has been good and positive growth.

Certainly many members of the nursing profession have been stimulated to think about their responsibilities in a wider sense than they had before. As for the organisations who number registered and enrolled nurses in their membership, their positions have been clarified. The Royal College of Nursing had declared itself against the use of withdrawal of labour as a weapon shortly before the statement was released. The Confederation of Health Service Employees and the National Union of Public Employees have since issued helpful documents to their memberships, providing guidance in this difficult area, and some guidelines against which to measure any proposed actions in a particular local situation. I welcome these documents for what they say on the subject, for the responsible attitudes which they encourage, and for the positive thought that obviously lies behind them. The period is one that has not only contained a debate of some genuine value but made a contribution to the nurse's understanding of what professional responsibility entails. Those with governmental or civil service responsibilities who where outside the debate, though doubtless watching it with interest, should recognise that those responsibilities include the need to operate in such a manner that the gap between the desirable and the achievable shrinks, and thus remove from professional nurses the temptation to assume that the ultimate weapon—withdrawal of labour—is the only effective weapon.

Are the recent trends in the professional disciplinary sphere or their implications good or bad? I can label three of the trends (or in the first case an established fact) as undoubtedly good:

1. the diminution in the number of cases being reported that are solely concerned with a nurse's personal life and have nothing to do with his or her professional life

2. more constructive kinds of cases are coming to the attention of the Council because members of the nursing profession are becoming more knowledgeable about and conscious of their personal professional responsibilities

3. a more informed public is aware that a case brought to the knowledge of the General Nursing Council for England and Wales by a private citizen will be subjected to exactly the same processes as those followed in cases brought by nurse managers.

Against that there are two trends that I label as bad:

a. a significant percentage of the growing number of cases (especially allegation cases) either result directly from or are affected vitally by the pressures and stress of an often grossly inadequate working situation

b. some cases indicate that, in certain situations, the extended role of the nurse has been introduced for the wrong reasons and in a manner that increases the burdens of already overburdened nursing staff.

Industrial action is not labelled good or bad, because it can take many forms. While some are undoubtedly bad, there may be circumstances in which a particular form of industrial action can be a positive, indeed, even a professionally responsible course to follow. I have also chosen to avoid labelling industrial action as good or bad because I hope that this particular new trend will rapidly become a thing of the past. Whether it does is dependent on a lot of people—not just the nurses who are at the sharp end of the business!

REFERENCES

Editorial (1979) The Rocky Path of Professionalism. *Nursing Times*, 2 August.

Editorial (1979) Grasping the GNC's Nettle. *Nursing Mirror*, 2 August.

10

What of the Future?

Change in the operation of the professional disciplinary process is inevitable, as is the type of caseload with which that process must deal, because the pressure, stress, risk and temptation of the world and of the nurses' workplace also change.

The history of the regulation of the nursing profession reveals that, at various stages since the 1919 Nurses Registration Act, the nursing councils have sought new statutory rules to enable alteration in some aspects of their professional disciplinary process. Had the Nurses, Midwives and Health Visitors Act not become law in 1979, further amendments to rules would have had to be made in an attempt to deal with some of the new and urgent problems faced by the responsible disciplinary bodies. One real test of this new act will be the measure of just how adequately any or all of these problems can be tackled.

The Nurses, Midwives and Health Visitors Act, 1979, provides for the regulation of the three professions through the professional disciplinary machinery of the new bodies it establishes. In common with the acts under which the present nursing and midwifery statutory bodies exist, this new act contains few words on the subject, leaving the bulk of the legal framework and procedures to be set down in rules which will require parliamentary approval in the form of statutory instruments. The relevant clauses of the new act are:

Introductory paragraph

> An Act to establish a Central Council for Nursing, Midwifery and Health Visiting, and National Boards for the four parts of the United Kingdom; to make new provision with respect to the education, training, *regulation and discipline of nurses, midwives and health visitors* and the maintenance of a single professional register; to amend an Act relating to the Central Council for Education and Training in Social Work; and for purposes connected with those matters (4th April 1979). [Italics mine.]

Section 2. Functions of the Central Council

Subclause 1
The principal functions of the Central Council shall be to establish and improve standards of training and *professional conduct* for nurses, midwives and health visitors.

Subclause 5
The powers of the Council shall include that of providing, in such manner as it thinks fit, advice for nurses, midwives and health visitors on standards of professional conduct.

Section 6. Functions of the National Boards

Subclause 1e
Carry out investigations of cases of alleged misconduct, with a view to proceedings before the Central Council or a committee of the Council for a person to be removed from the Register.

Section 12. Removal/restoration functions

1. The Central Council shall by rules determine circumstances in which, and the means by which:
(a) a person may, for misconduct or otherwise, be removed from the Register or a part of it, whether or not for a specified period;
(b) a person who has been removed from the Register or a part of it may be restored to it; and
(c) an entry in the Register may be removed, altered or restored.
2. Committees of the Council shall be constituted by the rules to hear and determine proceedings of a person's removal from, or restoration to, the Register or for the removal, alteration or restoration of any entry.
3. The committees shall be constituted from members of the Council; and the rules shall so provide that the members of a committee constituted to adjudicate upon the conduct of any person are selected with due regard to the professional field in which that person works.
4. The rules shall make provision as to the procedure to be followed, and the rules of evidence to be observed, in such proceedings, whether before the Council itself or before any committee so constituted, and for the proceedings to be in public except in such cases (if any) as the rules may specify.
5. Schedule 3 to this Act has effect with respect to the conduct of proceedings to which this section applies.

Section 13. Respondent's right of appeal

1. A person aggrieved by a decision to remove him [or her] from the Register, or to remove or alter any entry in respect of him [or her], may, within 3 months after the date on which notice of the decision is given to him [or her] by the Council, appeal to the appropriate Court; and on the appeal:

(a) the court may give such directions in the matter as it thinks proper, including directions as to the costs of the appeal; and
(b) the order of the court shall be final.
2. The appropriate court for the purposes of this section is the High Court, the Court of Session or the High Court in Northern Ireland, according as the appellant's ordinary place of residence is in England and Wales, Scotland or Northern Ireland at the time when notice of the decision is given.

Those parts of the act provide the legislative base, and on to them must be grafted the considerable volume of statutory rules which will provide the actual working machinery. The task of drafting those rules is a difficult, indeed even a dangerous one; it must be approached with care and without undue haste. What is most important is that the rule drafters take note of and retain all that is good in the processes of the five nursing and midwifery bodies (that are to be replaced by the new Central Council and National Boards), but must also take note of and, if possible within the terms of the act, prepare subordinate legislation which overcomes the present problems. The primary purpose of the new legislation, as with that it replaces, is the protection of the public. This has to be achieved (a) by ensuring that those who become registered have attained a suitable level of competence; (b) by maintaining records to show from whom the public might expect a competent, safe and caring service; and (c) by reinforcing that service through appropriate sanctions when failure is proved.

If protecting the vulnerable public is to be completed satisfactorily these are the 'problems' which have to be tackled. They are in some respects a restatement of points in Chapter 8, but are re-examined here because of their importance. In its professional disciplinary role, the Central Council for Nursing, Midwifery and Health Visiting will be regarded as either a success or failure against how it resolves these problems.

NEW CASES

Getting the right cases into the open and dealing with them

I indicated earlier that the reasons for the increase in the disciplinary caseload of the General Nursing Council for England and Wales are: (a) that more constructive kinds of case are now beginning to come to the surface and be reported, and (b) that this is at least to some extent a result of the strenuous attempts that Council has made to educate the members of the nursing profession to this aspect of their respon-

sibilities. The latter activity is one that was not placed on the Council
by the Act of Parliament under which it exists, but one which it has
voluntarily adopted (with an intensification of that activity in recent
years).

As one who has been heavily involved in such activity I at first
tended to be offended by that section of the act which requires the
Central Council to provide advice on standards of professional conduct. Why legislate for such an obvious function which the body for
which I have been privileged to work over the formative years of this
new act has been undertaking voluntarily? On reflection I decided
that subclause 5 of Section 2 is valuable, because it renders official the
need to make the professional practitioners conscious of their responsibilities. It clearly cannot be acceptable professional conduct to ignore
the wilfully reckless behaviour of a professional colleague. Subclause 5
of Section 2, through the encouragement it provides in this respect,
may well help to ensure that the more constructive kind of cases do
come to the attention of the Central Council so that it can fulfil its
responsibility to the public.

Dealing with cases without undue delay

Becoming aware of the right kind of cases is one thing, but actually
dealing with them in a relatively few weeks is quite another. It is
anomalous if the law that exists to protect the public itself stands in the
way of the achievement of that objective. That is to some degree,
however, what does happen and I suspect in some respects (though I
hope not all) may continue to happen under the terms of the new act.

What are these delays? How do they come about? Can they be
prevented in the future? I think I can answer the first two of those
questions. The answer to the third will lie in part with the rule drafters
and the new Central Council, but to some considerable degree it will lie
outside the Council's power to control or influence. Thinking first of
the present and the difficulties that exist, I can identify the following
points:

1. Delay before criminal trials at Crown Courts
The concern caused by long and seemingly increasing delays before
criminal trials at Crown Court could be illustrated in many ways, but
one story should suffice.

> A district nurse working in London was charged with a number of
> serious acts of theft from old people when she was visiting in their
> homes in the course of her duties. She pleaded not guilty in the
> Magistrates Court, and the case is to go to Crown Court for trial by

jury. She is suspended from duty by her employers, but takes up other nursing work through an agency. The police officer concerned telephoned to explain the circumstances, and to explain the evidence which they have, which appears very strong. He was expecting that, provided with such evidence, the Council would be able to suspend the nurse's right to practise, and was shocked to learn that this was not legally possible. More than a year has elapsed at the time of writing, and there is yet no sign of the case being scheduled for a hearing at Crown Court.

The past practice has been for the General Nursing Council for England and Wales to stand back and await the outcome of a criminal trial once charges have been laid against a nurse, and this was no great embarrassment when there were no significant delays in that process. Innocence must be assumed until guilt is proved. Now, however, the problem is extremely serious. The Council could deal with such matters as allegation cases if they became aware of them before criminal charges were laid (case 8 in Chapter 2 is an example of this). That means that it is possible to proceed to an early professional consideration of the allegations involved. If the allegations are proved and are considered to be misconduct, the right to practise can be taken from that nurse, if that is deemed to be the appropriate judgement. If that course of action is followed, instead of a criminal trial followed by a professional judgement on a finding of guilt, then while the public are protected from that person as a nurse, he or she will have avoided the judgement of society through the courts.

The statutory bodies are faced with a serious dilemma, but can anything be done about it under the new legislation? It seems surprising that our legislators, while carrying into the new act the previously existing clause which allows for the suspension of a midwife from practice, failed to allow for such a step to be taken in certain limited and justifiable circumstances for a nurse. It might be possible for something yet to be done about it under Section 12, subclause 1a, by the way in which rules are made. If Parliament allows such a control under the rules that at some future stage must come before them in a draft Statutory Instrument they could remedy what I see as an omission from the Nurses, Midwives and Health Visitors Act.

Until the situation changes this is a dilemma not only for the statutory bodies but for nurse managers. Faced with a particular set of circumstances (e.g., a psychiatric nurse who has physically abused patients) nurse managers must stop and decide what they want. Do they want a relatively quick professional judgement on that nurse's actions, with the possible removal of the right to practice, or do they want at some point in the future the punishment on behalf of society through the criminal courts, followed later still by a professional judgement?

2. *Getting cases heard once reported to the statutory bodies*

The present law under which the General Nursing Council for England and Wales operates requires certain procedures to be followed (see Chapters 4 to 6). The *shortest* time in which a case can go through the system from the initial report to the Disciplinary Committee decision is about 5 weeks. I emphasise shortest because of the present very serious problem in this respect.

The problem arose partly due to an increasing number of cases (especially time-consuming allegation cases) had to be dealt with by the same size committee as that used when the workload was much smaller. In early 1980 the delay between the Investigating Committee deciding that a case justifies a hearing before the Disciplinary Committee and that hearing taking place was a minimum of 3 months, but steadily increasing. When you add that to the probably long delay awaiting trial, or the sometimes several weeks or months of delay before a nurse manager brings a case to the attention of the Council, you can readily see that this is no way to protect the public.

It should not be assumed that the Council have done nothing about it. The frequency of Disciplinary Committee meetings has been steadily increased so that by Spring 1980 there were three (each of approximately 7 hours' duration) each month. The burden that this places on the committee members, all of whom have busy working lives, is enormous. In addition the Council successfully sought a change to the statutory rules to increase the size of the Disciplinary Committee (from twelve to sixteen) while leaving the quorum unchanged at six.

Does the new act make it possible to avoid this problem in the future? It may, but again the rule-making will be crucial. It has been the practice of the General Nursing Council for England and Wales to try to ensure that the twelve members who make up its Disciplinary Committee at any time include representatives of all nursing specialities, and that the Committee assembled to hear a particular case includes members with qualifications in the speciality concerned.

The problem becomes greater where the Central Council has to create a committee structure to perform this same function in respect of three professions. The relevant clause of the Nurses, Midwives and Health Visitors Act, 1979, states:

> The committees shall be constituted from members of the Council;
> and the rules shall so provide that the members of a committee

constituted to adjudicate upon the conduct of any person are selected with due regard to the professional field in which that person works.

This can be achieved through a two-committee structure: a Disciplinary Committee equivalent, which would be composed of all Central Council members who are *not* members of the Committee which must perform the equivalent function to the existing Investigating Committee. This would provide a large pool (perhaps as large as 35 members) from which to draw a committee that satisfies that clause. Another reason why the pool should be large enough to spread the burden widely is that more than half the Central Council members will also be members of National Boards and have responsibilities at that level as well. The logistical difficulties are considerable, but not insoluble.

3. *Getting a consumer voice heard in the professional disciplinary process*

The statutory rules made under the terms of the Nurses Act, 1969, determine the professional disciplinary process of the General Nursing Council for England and Wales. Significantly, they include a rule which requires that at least two of the sixteen members of the Disciplinary Committee must not be nurses. This rule has been made, although the Nurses Act contains nothing that requires it.

The intention of this rule, I assumed, was to ensure that while peer judgement is essential in determining a nurse's appropriateness to practise the public should also be represented if the law exists for their protection. If that was the intention I would applaud it. The number from whom to draw the non-nurse representatives, however, is small; it is, therefore, difficult to ensure that there is 'public' representation. Often these places have been filled by doctors who, although their contribution is excellent, hardly bring the objectivity to the task that I think was intended. In addition to that the existing rule, while requiring two (at least) non-nurse Council members to be included in the Committee, does not insist that any of them be part of the particular group (minimum six) assembled to hear a particular case.

Some other statutory bodies for the health professions obtain their non-nurse members for their Disciplinary Committee by direct appointment of members of the public to that Committee rather than limiting the opportunity to Council members. Unfortunately, this is precluded by the opening words of Section 12, subclause 3 of the act: 'The committees shall be so constituted *from members of the Council*'. Perhaps my final suggestion under the previous heading would help to provide the answer.

RESTORATION TO THE REGISTER OR ROLL OF NURSES

When I speak to audiences of nurses and ask them to consider a case study about a restoration application, and then to answer the question Would you restore this person to the Register?, they tend to ask if the person must have some retraining to bring them up to date before taking up employment as a registered nurse. The answer is No. This aspect of the system is regarded by the participants as unsafe. Is it any less safe to allow a nurse to have a 15-year period away from nursing and then return to the full role of a registered nurse without any sort of refresher course, or (as has recently happened) for a person having become eligible to register to delay application for registration for over 20 years?

I do agree that some form of refresher or further training is desirable for those who are restored after a substantial gap, but I am convinced that it would be unreasonable to single them out. It is the whole question of nurses returning to practise after a substantial break (whatever the reason) that must be tackled.

What of the different features that are introduced by the new act, and the new opportunities that it provides? There are, I suggest, just two points to make that have not been ventilated under my consideration of present problems.

The first concerns the procedures that will have to be prepared in accordance with statutory rules and consequential administrative policies. The original concept of the four National Boards for the countries of the United Kingdom was that they would be National Education Boards, with the responsibilities that went with that title. Somewhere along the way, however, the idea changed so that when the bill (that with some amendment became the Nurses, Midwives and Health Visitors Act) was published the word *education* had been dropped from the title, and just one function that was not associated with the broad subject of nursing, midwifery and health visiting education and training was inserted. It is found in Section 6, subclause 1e and reads:

> Carry out investigations of alleged misconduct, with a view to proceedings before the Central Council or a committee of the Council for a person to be removed from the Register.

What does that mean? Since it uses the word *alleged* I take it to mean that any *allegations* brought to the attention of a National Board must be investigated by an appropriate officer and solicitor for that Board, considered by a Board committee, and that they must decide if such an *allegation* case is considered to justify a hearing. I also take it to mean that, since Section 12, subclause 2 of the act requires that 'Committees' (in the plural) be constituted to hear and determine proceedings at Central Council, what I have previously described as 'conviction cases' from any of the four countries will go straight to the Central Council and, after obtaining the nurses' comments and the like, will go for a preliminary assessment to a sieving committee.

If these are correct conclusions, they add still further to the previously described major logistical problems, as no National Board member who participates in a preliminary committee consideration of an allegation case should then participate in the hearing conducted by the appropriate committee of the Central Council. Probably the only safe course to pursue would be for the appropriate committee of the National Board to be drawn from among those of its members who are not also members of the Central Council.

The second point, though contained in only two words, is of great significance. The present law limits the Council to removing from the Register or Roll only those nurses who have done something culpable and have subsequently been found guilty of professional misconduct. It is not possible to 'resign' from the Register, no matter how inadequate and unsafe a practitioner you may consider yourself. This need not necessarily be so in the future. Whereas the outgoing law, in its section on removal from the Register refers to established misconduct as the only prerequisite to possible removal, the new act refers to the fact that a person may 'for misconduct *or otherwise*, be removed from the Register or a part of it'. Those two words (italics mine) provide the future statutory bodies with a tremendous challenge and a tremendous opportunity. The challenge and the opportunity are to improve still further the protection of the public, while assisting the rehabilitation of members of the nursing profession *before they are guilty of some culpable act*.

What use will the Central Council make of this opportunity? Certainly many nurses who become the subject of disciplinary cases are sick people rather than bad people, but have gone on until they do something wrong. Can that become a thing of the past?

What does it cost to protect the public in this way? Who pays? are questions which I face regularly. The short answer in the nursing profession is that, though the purpose of the law is the protection of the public, it is the profession that pays through the fees of its members. In 1978/79 it needed the registration and enrolment fees of nearly 2,700 nurses to meet the cost of that year's professional disciplinary work.

Ironically, although the outgoing midwifery legislation is also about the protection of the public it comes to the conclusion that the costs of the statutory midwifery body be met from public funds. Now these two professions, and the health visiting profession, come together under the new legislation which view will prevail? Section 10 of the Nurses, Midwives and Health Visitors Act refers to the one professional register and its various parts; both here and in Section 11 reference is made to 'such fee as may be required by rules'. It would therefore be possible to have no fees. Which way will the rule makers jump, and will the responsible ministers agree with them? Surely it will not be possible for nurses to go on paying fees and midwives not when those different professional qualifications are parts of the same single professional register? If consistency is to be introduced does that mean that midwives will have to pay fees when they have not done so before?

The professional disciplinary responsibilities of the new bodies are important, as are their other functions. Important principles are at stake, but the questions have yet to be answered!

So my look towards the future with its challenges, opportunities and risks concludes. However, I cannot bring my book to a conclusion without iterating the conviction I hold that any specially educated occupational group, if it is to be worthy of the title Profession, must readily accept the responsibility of regulating itself. It must do this, not to maintain the purity of the profession, or for self-aggrandizement, but to protect the public. This is part of our professional heritage. We have heavy responsibility to our professional predecessors, to ensure that their hard won victories in achieving not only the registration of nurses but the self-regulation of their profession do not go for nought. But we also have a responsibility to hand on a profession in good order. If we are to succeed in that aim it needs to be a profession that continues to oppose poor standards and promote what is good; it needs to be a profession that continues to respond to the increasingly technical demands made on it, yet without forsaking those essential qualities of care, kindness and compassion; it needs to be a profession made up of people who are professionals in their own right and conscious of the responsibilities that they bear for their standards of patient care, the settings in which patients are cared for, and not least for their colleagues. I hope that this book will make some contribution to the acceptance of that responsibility.

Appendix A

Case Studies on Professional Responsibility and the Regulation of the Nursing Profession

By now the reader should have a reasonable understanding of the way in which the nursing profession regulates itself through the professional disciplinary process. For the individual or group desiring to go further into the subject and to stimulate some discussion regarding professional responsibility, I set out a number of extra case studies. Having used these and others like them in study days and seminars around Great Britain I am convinced that nurses identify easily with the questions raised. Many tell me that having participated in such events, they returned to their wards or departments with greater recognition of the hazards to be found there, and of their responsibilities. May this also be the experience of those who use this Appendix.

The cases, like those preceding, are based directly on cases considered since 1976 by the relevant committees of the General Nursing Council for England and Wales, and are truncated only to present in a few paragraphs, what may have emerged in a public hearing over several hours.

The decisions made by the committees on these cases, and those in the text, together with some comments, are given in Appendix B. I suggest reference to that section be made only after a case has been considered and discussed. To facilitate reference, there is a Table of Cases on page 155. Please remember that there are no right or wrong answers in this exercise. Follow the structure and composition of the real committees for your study or seminar committees, with each member participating from the background of his or her own knowledge and experience.

CASE A1. DISCIPLINARY COMMITTEE—CONVICTION

A 27-year-old SRN appeared before the Disciplinary Committee of the General Nursing Council for England and Wales following an appearance in a

115

Magistrates Court where she had pleaded guilty to stealing a quantity of pentazocine (Fortral) ampoules and syringes from the hospital in which she had been employed for just a few months. Her employment had been terminated as a result.

She attended the Disciplinary Committee with her father and a family friend. The documents assembled for that occasion included not only those that confirmed the conviction but also a letter from her father sent to the Investigating Committee and a medical report. The nurse had already established a useful relationship with one of the professional social workers from the Nurses Welfare Service, and the Committee were able to receive a report from that source at the appropriate stage of the hearing.

The medical report indicated a 6-year history of dyspepsia, epigastric pain and bleeding, there being both medical treatment and surgical interventions for vagotomy, hiatus hernia, cholecystectomy, to which could be added frequent endoscopy and other investigations. On two occasions the situation was further complicated by occurrences of deep vein thrombosis. Investigations were in hand at the time of the hearing. The consultant who wrote the medical report felt that the past extensive investigations had not always led to satisfactory treatment. He also stated his opinion that intramuscular Fortral had been necessary for the relief of her pain.

The nurse's father referred to the fact that the drug which led to her conviction was that which various doctors had given her in the past for self-injection, and that throughout this 6-year period of frequent illness she had done her best to sustain her career.

In answer to the Committee's questions she indicated that she was still on oral Fortral, which she was taking about twice a day. She felt that she had been placed in an impossible position which prevented her from going to her new GP for assistance because he was also the hospital's occupational health doctor, and she felt that for him to become aware of a recurrence of her problem may well lead to her losing the nursing post into which she had only recently moved. She told the Committee that she did not intend to seek nursing employment until her doctors had assured her that she was well enough.

The welfare adviser's report indicated that, when applying for the nursing post in which the incident occurred, she had not felt able to disclose the full extent of her health problems as it would mean she did not get the chance to re-establish herself in nursing. He had ascertained that the court case had been heavily reported in the local papers, and on regional television news, all of which had a shattering effect, increased her level of anxiety, and so exacerbated her symptoms. He felt that she was a pleasant, caring person who had shown courage in the face of serious and long-standing illness, and that she now realised that her attempt to treat herself (even though with the drug which had so often been prescribed for her in the past) was unwise. For their part, the Committee felt concern that it was still the same analgesic that she was receiving from the family GP.

The Disciplinary Committee considered her offence to be misconduct. Which of the three decisions open to them would you consider appropriate in this case?

CASE A2. DISCIPLINARY COMMITTEE—CONVICTION

The General Nursing Council for England and Wales received a letter from a nurse manager about an SRN, RMN, aged 41 years, who had been dismissed from his post as a nursing officer in a special home for disabled people following the conviction referred to in the local paper from which the nurse manager enclosed a cutting, headed 'Ex-nurse pocketed charity's money'. The police confirmed the conviction shortly after this letter was received. The gist of the newspaper report, substantially confirmed by the notice of the conviction, was that he had obtained money from a charity purporting that it was for patients and then used it himself and that he had obtained meat and eggs from a butcher by purporting that they were for the home when they were for his own use.

The Investigating Committee had no more information than that, since he had not replied to the Council's letter inviting any explanation he might wish to offer. That Committee forwarded the case for a disciplinary hearing. Some days before the hearing date, having received the formal notice and the letter explaining his rights of attendance, representation, the nurse telephoned to say he would not be attending as the outcome was obvious. He clearly felt that the Council had never before had to deal with anyone as bad as he. He was told again of the importance of attendance, the point that the matter was not prejudged being again strongly emphasised. At the end of that discussion the officer concerned had no clear idea of whether he would attend.

Obviously he thought about it further and on the day he did attend without any representation. He had by then written a letter for the Committee which was copied for all members and which formed the basis of their subsequent questions. In that letter he referred again to his awful crime, and explained the complicated domestic background against which it was set. For both him and his wife this was a second marriage, she having two daughters by the first marriage. There came a time when the elder daughter wished to live with her father; to try to stop her the wife engaged in lavish spending on clothes, shoes, cosmetics.

Meanwhile the nurse was working away from home, and planning to move the family to his new area. Each time he came home his wife was depressed and complaining, but on one special occasion he came home for a week's holiday to find the position even worse than usual—there was no food in the house, no money in the bank, mountainous debts, demand notices for various sums with threats of court action, the telephone cut off, and gas/electricity supplies about to be cut off—and all to prevent the daughter's return to her father! He attempted to borrow money from family and friends, but was refused because his wife had already borrowed from them and the money had not been repaid.

In answer to the Committee's question about his present situation, he explained that he was unemployed for a few weeks, and then obtained work in a factory, in addition to which he was working through a nursing agency to earn extra money so as to speedily make restitution. By the time of the hearing he had repaid almost half the money. The Committee were impressed by the man and his determination to work very hard to redeem the situation. The elder daughter had now left home to live with her grandparents, his wife had returned to work as a secretary, the marriage was more stable financially and emotionally. His total working week (factory, plus nursing agency work at weekends, days off) was about 80 hours, at which rate he would clear his debt in 2 further months. He was hoping to return to full-time geriatric nursing in the Health Service.

The Committee considered the offences misconduct. Which of the three available decisions would you choose?

CASE A3. DISCIPLINARY COMMITTEE—CONVICTION

A 25-year-old SRN appeared before the Disciplinary Committee of the General Nursing Council for England and Wales as a result of a conviction (on her own plea of guilty) in a Magistrates Court for the theft of cash, foreign currency, and a radio/cassette player from private patients in the hospital where she had been employed, a raincoat from a colleague, and some penicillin tablets from the hospital. The court imposed a Community Service Order. Her employment had been terminated.

At the Disciplinary Committee some months later the nurse was present but not represented. The documents before the Committee included the nurse's letter to the Investigating Committee, a copy of the medical report that had been prepared for the court (who initially remanded her on bail for the purpose of receiving this), and an up-to-date medical report prepared for the Committee. At the appropriate stage the Committee received not only a welfare report but (through the welfare adviser) a report from the community service organiser and a report from the senior partner in a large dental practice for which she was then working.

The first medical report indicated that at the time of the incident, it appeared that she had become depressed and consequently beset with sleep disturbance and apathy, and that whereas many temporarily isolated women would make a poor attempt at suicide to draw attention, she stole as her cry for help. The consultant had been impressed with the fact that once it had all come into the open she had been able to talk to various counsellors and was much less tense. In the second and up-dating report written for the benefit of the Committee the consultant indicated that he had continued to see her and that she had recovered from her transient depressive illness. He was pleased that she had been able to talk her problems through with boyfriend, family, and others, and he felt no concern at the prospect of her returning to nursing.

The community service order organiser expressed her delight that the nurse had shown total commitment to the work required by the order and proved to be one of the most reliable people she had met. Because of her efforts new openings had been created for community service in the future, and some other offenders helpfully introduced to their duties.

Her dentist employers, with full knowledge of the facts, said how conscientious and capable they had found her, and how mature her attitudes. They had made her manageress of their multiple unit surgery, giving her responsibility for ordering stock and for patients' payments.

The welfare adviser, from the basis of good contact, indicated how significant it was that, having failed her midwifery examination for the second time, she came to a post in a teaching hospital where she felt that all around her were much more able than herself. This feeling of diappointment and inadequacy coincided with the death of her grandmother (for whom she had great affection), and concern about her developing relationship with a man whose two previous marriages had ended in divorce.

Looking back on the events, the nurse told the Committee that it was as if someone else was committing the offences and that she was looking on. She was obviously relieved to be caught, and grateful for the understanding and help she had since received. Everything pointed to the fact that this was totally out of character and that she was a kind, caring and (in spite of failing her midwifery examination) competent nurse. Her responses to the Committee's questions were very honest and open, and left them in no doubt that she was very sorry, and fully realised the significance of her actions.

The Committee considered the matters to be professional misconduct. Which of the available decisions would you have chosen?

CASE A4. DISCIPLINARY COMMITTEE—ALLEGATION

A 30-year-old SRN and a 34-year-old SEN became the subject of a joint hearing before the Disciplinary Committee of the General Nursing Council for England and Wales as a result of allegations brought by a divisional nursing officer that they had been fighting on duty. The ward in question was a female surgical/gynaecological ward, and the incident happened at approx. 9:15 P.M. between two nurses whose night duty had commenced at 8:00 P.M.

The SEN was a direct employee of the authority, and she had worked regularly on this ward for some months. The SRN was a nurse supplied by an agency; she had been working in this hospital for some weeks, and had worked on this particular ward on two or three occasions. (As the hearing emerged, that there was no clear policy as to which nurse would be 'in charge' in such a situation became steadily more significant.) On this night the agency nurse had reported to the nursing officer and had been sent to take charge of the ward in question for the night.

From the time of her arrival on the ward the SEN seemed to resent that she was not in charge on her own ward, and was clearly hostile in her attitude towards the SRN. Evidence to this effect was given by an auxiliary from the same ward, and another SEN from an adjacent ward who had come to obtain some intravenous fluids. The first of them, in her evidence, described the general feeling of animosity and unease that was created, and the exchange of verbal insults she heard, mostly by the SEN and directed at the SRN. The second (the other SEN) told how she had come along the ward corridor off which ran a number of single and double side rooms for patients. She explained that the SRN was attempting to administer medication from the trolley, but was being harangued by the SEN, who was clearly upset about something and regarded it as the fault of the SRN.

According to the latter witness the situation exploded when the SRN reacted by speaking offensive words to the SEN, who then physically attacked her, causing the trolley to crash against the wall and various tablets and bottles to fall to the floor by the open door of a single room in which a patient was recovering from an operation earlier that day. The SRN took action to defend herself, and the two wrestled in the doorway, and eventually were carried by their own impetus into the patient's room.

The patient was the remaining witness. She had returned to the ward at about 1:30 P.M. following a hysterectomy, and had been given an injection during the afternoon. She described how she was wakened from a dozing state by a 'scrunching noise', which was presumably that of nurses' feet on tablets and bottles. She then realised that there were two nurses violently fighting in her room, and worried as the ebb and flow of the fight sometimes brought them near to falling on her bed, and even on to her operation wound. She regarded the large nurse (the SEN) as the aggressor, and thought the other was simply doing her best to defend herself.

In her evidence the SRN admitted calling the SEN a 'hog', after which she was subjected to a violent attack. The SEN in evidence said that the word *hog* had been used against her but with an even more offensive adjective. She also claimed that it had not happened as described and that she was only acting in self-defence.

The Committee found the allegations true, and accepted that the SEN was the aggressor, but felt that the SRN had helped to provoke the situation. They considered the actions of both nurses to be professional misconduct. Would you have made that decision? If so, which of the three available decisions would you then have made?

CASE A5. DISCIPLINARY COMMITTEE—CONVICTION

A district nursing officer alerted the senior welfare adviser of the Nurses Welfare Service about a 29-year-old sister of a medical ward in a large district general hospital. She had admitted taking Omnopon from the ward stock and getting student nurses to inject her with the drug on the pretext that she was undergoing prescribed hormone treatment. In addition to notifying the Council officially about the incident, the district nursing officer felt that the welfare service should be involved at an early stage because she suspected the sister (whom she had dismissed from employment) was under severe emotional stress.

An immediate offer of help was made in writing to the sister. This she accepted and when the senior welfare adviser went to visit her he found her in a very depressed state as a result of a breakdown in her matrimonial relationship, coupled with rejection by her father. She impressed him as an intelligent, articulate girl who set herself very high standards of patient care and took a great pride in her work. She felt unable to admit to anyone how she was feeling and resorted to taking Omnopon.

Having been involved from the outset, the senior welfare adviser was able to help her work through her depression, liaise with her psychiatrist, advise her about legal aid for the forthcoming court case, refer her to the local probation and after-care service, and prepare her for the eventual hearing of her case by the Disciplinary Committee of the General Nursing Council.

She was given a conditional discharge by the court because of the quality of all-round support she receiving. Three months later, the case was considered by the Disciplinary Committee. Meanwhile, with the client's consent, the senior welfare adviser had obtained a psychiatric report and a social enquiry report which were presented to the Committee. She was accompanied by her husband (with whom she was by then reconciled) and her former senior nursing officer, who had been enormously supportive from the outset. Though, still somewhat depressed and not unnaturally extremely apprehensive about the hearing, she presented well to the Committee. The psychiatrist expressed the view that there was no drug dependence and that she was not suffering from any major psychiatric illness.

If you had been a member of the Disciplinary Committee which of the following decisions would you have made?

a. caution
b. postponed judgement
c. removal from the Register

CASE A6. DISCIPLINARY COMMITTEE—ALLEGATION

A 44-year-old SRN appeared before the Disciplinary Committee charged with misappropriating pethidine for her own use which she admitted. This case came to light when she had been working at a hospital as an agency staff nurse. The police were involved but decided not to prosecute; she was given an official police caution instead.

The senior welfare adviser made an offer of help to her early in the development of the case. She was quick to respond, and in fact was very much in need of intensive support in the 2 months' build-up to the disciplinary hearing. By careful planning it was possible to arrange for her case to be considered by the Disciplinary Committee of the Central Midwives Board (she is also a midwife) and of the General Nursing Council on the same day.

She had been working two nights a week through an agency for several years thereby carrying her responsibilities towards her family (she has two children aged 6 and 4) and at the same time pursuing her professional career. The immediate contributory cause of her helping herself to pethidine from the ward stock was the pain she was suffering as a result of burning her feet on a hot water bottle. She had not sought medical help at the time because she was very involved in preparations for Christmas. Meanwhile, the pain became increasingly more severe and it was while she was in this state that she took the pethidine. When she eventually consulted her doctor she was told that she was suffering from second degree burns and that a period of hospitalisation was desirable. She was allowed home, however, on condition that she rested.

In his report to the Committee the senior welfare adviser explained that there were problems in the matrimonial relationship which had been under severe strain for some considerable time. Communication was a very real difficulty both in the client's relationship with her husband and with her mother, who lived in an adjacent bungalow. Isolation was identified as another problem through her geographical location, job and temperament.

The client attended the hearing on her own. The senior welfare adviser presented a social background report; a psychiatric report was also available. She presented well and it was obvious that her health had improved significantly and that she was making full use of all the support available to her.

An additional and important factor was that the divisional nursing officer with responsibility for the general hospital in which the incident occurred (and in which this nurse had been working fairly regularly for some months) came to the hearing and told the Committee how kind and competent this nurse was, and how high her standards of care were. This is most unusual when the case concerns an agency nurse.

Which of the three decisions would you have made and why?

CASE A7. INVESTIGATING COMMITTEE—CONVICTION

A state enrolled nurse, aged 26 years, was convicted of shoplifting as a result of which she was cautioned by letter by the Investigating Committee of the General Nursing Council for England and Wales. At the time she had been married for 5 years, and had a 4-year-old daughter.

For the past 4 years her husband had treated her violently and she has now obtained an injunction banning him from going near her, the child or the matrimonial home. Although her husband is supposed to pay maintenance for her and the child, he has refused to do so. The nurse works during the week as an accounts clerk and does agency nursing at the weekend.

This nurse, however, has now appeared in court again, this time for the theft of a few small items of hospital property—crepe bandages, Elastoplast, antiseptic ointment. The theft came to light when the police were called to a domestic dispute and her husband insisted they search the house for stolen property. The nurse admits she stole the items but says it was all taken about 2 years ago to provide first aid equipment for her husband's football team.

This is the second time the General Nursing Council has been asked to consider her dishonesty. What do you think the Investigating Committee should decide this time? They can say that it:

a. is of no concern to the Council *or*

b. is of concern but can be dealt with by a letter of caution and counsel *or*

c. justifies a hearing before the Disciplinary Committee

CASE A8. DISCIPLINARY COMMITTEE—ALLEGATION

A 31-year-old SRN, employed by an Area Health Authority as a night community nurse in an inner city area, appeared before the Disciplinary Committee of the General Nursing Council for England and Wales to face charges that she failed to visit a patient, and made a false entry in the report book purporting to have made such a visit.

The Committee heard that the nurse had major difficulties in her personal life in that she had a husband who drank very heavily as a result of which the financial burden of supporting the family (they had an 8-year-old daughter) fell almost entirely on her. Apparently just before leaving to go on duty that night there had been something of a scene; she left the house not only feeling tired and unhappy but fearful for her daughter's safety, as her husband (under the influence of his usual and costly alcohol intake) was in a rather violent mood.

On her arrival at the patient's address the nurse was, therefore, feeling ill at ease. She got out of her car and made to approach the patient's flat which entailed going down a narrow passage. At the entrance to that passage there were two men who were obviously quite drunk and in a boisterous and threatening mood. The nurse explained that, after coming from a similar scene at home, she felt too distressed and frightened to risk trying to force her way past them to visit the patient. She returned to her car to make other calls. About an hour later she returned to try again, only to find the men again obstructing her path. She then took the step which in retrospect she realised was terribly wrong. She did not call her senior officer to indicate what had happened but made a false entry in the records.

At the hearing the nurse was represented by a full-time officer of her trade union. She was distressed as she recalled the events of that night, and was obviously ashamed that she had failed her patient, who, without the normal assistance to return to bed, was found still in her chair in the morning by the day community nurse who called to get her up.

It emerged in evidence that it was the normal practice for night nurses in this area to work in pairs, but on this night there was a shortage of staff so she was alone. It was explained that in the event of difficulty she should have contacted the nursing officer in charge of the local hospital who would have arranged for a member of the hospital staff to come and assist her, this being the local arrangement. (The Committee wondered if the hospital staff was adequate to allow that to happen without unreasonably reducing patient cover.) The nurse concerned was not aware of that arrangement until it was referred to in evidence. She said that had she been able to think rationally about the position she would have called the police to assist her gain admission.

On the basis of her recognised competence and normal high standards, and the evidence of her good work record since she commenced nursing at the age of 18 years, she had not been dismissed from her employment as a night community nurse. The Committee learnt that her husband had accepted that he had a drink problem and was attending Alcoholics Anonymous, and that the nurse was hopeful that her personal life might now become easier.

If you were a member of the Disciplinary Committee would you consider this nurse's action on that night Professional Misconduct? If so, would you then:

a. administer a caution but take no further action *or*
b. postpone judgement for a stated period *or*
c. remove the nurse's name from the Register

CASE A9. DISCIPLINARY COMMITTEE—ALLEGATION

A 33-year-old SRN appeared before the Disciplinary Committee of the General Nursing Council for England and Wales where she admitted allegations that, on two occasions, she had been unfit for duty when on duty due to alcohol. Because of her admission it was not necessary to call the witnesses to give evidence, but the Committee were given the details of the incidents.

The first incident occurred just a few weeks after she had commenced employment in a part-time capacity at the hospital where she had trained, and in which she had subsequently worked to her employer's great satisfaction. She presented herself for night duty and began to go about her work, but it was quickly observed that her behaviour was bizarre, her gestures exaggerated, her speech slurred, and her breath smelling of alcohol. When questioned she explained the position as being solely due to the glass or two of wine she had taken with her evening meal, which must have potentiated the effect of the Distalgesic she was taking for a back problem. Her explanation was in part accepted, but she was formally warned about the consequences of such actions.

However on a day 10 weeks later she again presented herself on duty in a condition that immediately drew attention. Her clothing was untidy which was not normal, she had extreme difficulty in making her hands perform the functions she intended, she was weepy, her speech rapidly became slurred and her eyes glazed. On this occasion it was suggested to her that she had a serious drink problem, and she agreed and spoke of the ill effect it was having on the lives of herself, her husband, and their two children. She agreed to be seen by a doctor, and he involved a psychiatrist, through whose intervention she became a patient of a specialist alcohol dependence unit. She was dismissed from her employment.

The hearing before the Disciplinary Committee took place several months after the second incident; she in the meantime had continued to receive treatment for her alcoholism. The reports from her psychiatrist confirmed that her problem had been very deep, that she had been working very hard to cooperate with the treatment, and that though considerable progress had been achieved there was yet no cause for complacency. She certainly seemed willing to accept her psychiatrist's advice which was to the effect that she should not contemplate returning to nursing employment until both he and her general practitioner thought it reasonable to do so.

As indicated earlier, the nurse had trained in the hospital where these incidents subsequently occurred. She had been the model student achieving consistently good results for all her theoretical work, high distinction in examinations, much admiration for her practical ability, and finally the Gold Medal for her year. She had subsequently worked as staff nurse and sister before leaving due to pregnancy, and returned for 2 years in a part-time capacity until another pregnancy. It was clear at each departure that they would re-employ her without hesitation, and that they subsequently did, but only to discover that she was now a nurse with a problem of some magnitude.

As a member of the Disciplinary Committee would you consider her admitted unfitness on duty to be professional misconduct? If so, which of the available decisions would you choose? You can:

a. administer a caution but take no other action *or*

b. postpone judgement for a stated period *or*

c. remove the nurse's name from the Register of Nurses

CASE A10. DISCIPLINARY COMMITTEE—ALLEGATION

A report was received concerning an SRN, aged 33 years, who had been dismissed from her post after admitting she administered Valium (which had not been prescribed) intravenously to a patient on three separate occasions. She had been employed as a nursing officer in charge of the nursing services of a large general hospital on night duty for several months.

She had trained as an SRN through a shortened course for existing graduates, having first worked in other spheres of activity for several years. Subsequent to becoming registered she had made rapid progress in her career, leading to her appointment as a nursing officer.

The case was put before the Investigating Committee who decided that it justified a hearing before the Disciplinary Committee. The circumstances were as follows: on the night that the incident occurred the nurse went to the private patients' ward. While she was on that ward she noticed that a patient was awake and appeared very restless and agitated. The nurse told the ward nurse that she thought that the patient should have an intravenous injection of Valium. The ward nurse said that the patient was written up for an intramuscular injection of Valium and that he had already been given it. The nursing officer decided that the patient should still be given some intravenous Valium, which she herself administered, because she felt that he might otherwise do himself harm. (The patient was a former member of the hospital staff.)

The nursing officer returned to the ward on two further occasions (at approximately hourly intervals) to see if the patient had settled down, but he was still in the same condition, so on each occasion she gave him another injection of Valium intravenously. On no occasion was a call made to any of the medical staff, either before or after the administration of the drug.

In her previous employment (elsewhere in the country) as a sister in a renal dialysis unit she had been one of the nursing staff authorised to give intravenous injections. It became clear that, in that employment, she was much respected by the medical staff for her wide knowledge, and in consequence was encouraged by them to perform certain clinical procedures outside her normal 'extended' role. In her period of employment as a nursing officer, because of her previous experience, she had been appointed to a working party in the health district which was to commence consideration of the extending clinical role of the nurse with particular reference to the administration of prescribed intravenous injections, but it had not met at the time of the incident.

The nurse had apparently been under a considerable amount of stress prior to the incident. There had been a series of family problems worrying her and also she had only recently rerurned to nursing duties after recovering from an illness herself.

If you had been a member of the Disciplinary Committee, which of the three available decisions would you have made in respect of her professional status?

CASE A11. DISCIPLINARY COMMITTEE—CONVICTION

A state enrolled nurse (on only the part of the Roll for Mental Nurses) appeared before the Disciplinary Committee, having been sent to prison for $2\frac{1}{2}$ years.

The incident occurred late in the evening outside the social club of the large psychiatric hospital where the nurse (and the other nurse who was the injured party) worked and resided. Certainly a substantial amount of alcohol had been consumed.

The prosecution case in court (which was the view that prevailed) had been that this nurse had come out of the club and launched an unprovoked attack with the glass he was carrying, and which he first broke for the purpose. The defence was that the injured person and his friends had been taunting and provoking the nurse, particularly about his protective relationship with an Indian girl (he was Malaysian) who had formerly been the girlfriend of the aggrieved who (it was said) had treated her badly and subsequently subjected her to continuous harassment.

It was not denied that there had been an assault, but it was said that it was a response to great provocation by the group who had gathered outside the club to wait for this nurse. He claimed that he was taking the empty glass with him to a party in one of the hospital houses, and that he had to defend himself when attacked and it accidentally broke and caused the injuries, for which he was very sorry.

The facial lacerations sustained required 38 sutures, and there were less serious lacerations on the arms. During the course of their investigation the police found the nurse to be in possession of a small quantity of Valium tablets in an envelope for which he could not account, so he was also convicted of possessing those drugs illegally.

This man claimed that he was not violent, and that nothing would have occurred if the girl had not been harassed, if he had not been provoked, and if the alcohol had not impaired his self-control. He seemed genuinely sorry. The fact remained, however, that he had been found guilty of 'wounding with intent'.

It was a conviction case. Would you consider that conviction to be professional misconduct?

If Yes, which of the three available decisions would you consider appropriate? You can:

a. administer a caution but take no further action *or*
b. postpone judgement for a period of time *or*
c. remove the nurse's name from the Roll of Nurses

CASE A12. DISCIPLINARY COMMITTEE—ALLEGATION

A divisional nursing officer for a large mental handicap division brought to the Council allegations concerning an RNMS aged 31 years.

It was alleged that the woman (who had been in the employment of the particular hospital for 11 years) had hit a child on the head with her shoe, and that she had submitted an accident form which misrepresented the facts as they subsequently emerged.

At the Disciplinary Committee the first witness was a nursing assistant (an intelligent young married woman who had been employed for 9 months). She was in charge of a ward for active mentally handicapped children at night and had been told to keep a special eye on a boy called Tommy. He began to play up and as she was anxious about the situation, and this was the first time she had been on this ward, she went to the adjacent ward to ask the trained nurse there for guidance. The nurse (the subject of the case) went to the nursing assistant's ward half an hour later, and helped her to cope with the situation and put the children to bed. The last was a boy named Philip. Shortly after this Philip got out of bed (which he had wet) and stripped it. The witness alleged that the nurse concerned took hold of Philip, smacked him on the face and body with the palm of her hand about 12 times, and then took her right shoe off. With that shoe she struck Philip a number of blows; one was a hard blow on top of the head. Philip then broke free and ran to hide behind a locker. The witness comforted the child and found that his face was covered with blood. The nurse took Philip to the bathroom, bathed his face, and located the cut. The nurse then said to the witness that she would have to report the matter, but it would be better to say that the child cut his head on the locker. She asked the witness to cover her if she said that. The witness was relatively inexperienced, and at first said that she would.

The doctor came and treated the wound. He signed the accident report on which it was stated that Philip had fallen and hit the corner of the locker. The witness thought the matter over, and when she was next on duty (4 days later) she reported the incident.

The second witness was the doctor (a registrar). He said that at about 10:30 P.M. he received a call from the ward and went as requested. Philip was brought to him and he found that there was a jagged laceration on the top of his head. This jagged wound was said to be about 4 cm long. He cleaned the wound, sutured it and applied a dressing. He then completed the partly filled accident form. The third witness was the divisional nursing officer. He gave evidence that having received a report from the nursing assistant, he interviewed the nurse in the presence of her union representative. The nurse admitted that she had contacted the patient with her shoe, but insisted that she had not struck the patient. He was told that she took the new shoe off because it was hurting her, and Philip rubbed his head against it. She admitted that she had submitted a false accident form. In consequence, the divisional nursing officer dismissed the nurse concerned, though in this evidence he did confirm that she had been in the employment of his division (as student and trained nurse) for 11 years, and there had been no previous cause for concern.

In her evidence the nurse insisted that she had taken her shoe off because it was hurting her, and that while she had it in her hand Philip ran into her and rubbed his head against the heel. She admitted that the evidence concerning the cover-up was true and that the accident report was false, but she said that she had submitted false particulars as she was 'shocked at what I had accidentally caused and I panicked'. She argued that never had she ever either knowingly or accidentally caused harm to a patient.

The Committee were satisfied that the allegations were proved, and that the facts constituted professional misconduct.

See yourself as the Disciplinary Committee. On the evidence would you have come to the same conclusion as the Disciplinary Committee? If Yes, what decision of the available three would you then have made about this registered nurse?

CASE A13. DISCIPLINARY COMMITTEE—ALLEGATION

A 28-year-old ward sister (the senior of two on the ward) appeared before the Disciplinary Committee to answer charges arising from an incident concerning one patient in her surgical ward.

On the day she returned from holiday, and while still becoming aware of the patients now occupying the ward, she was summoned urgently to the operating theatre to speak to a consultant surgeon about a patient she personally had not met. It was this discussion and the actions that followed that led to the allegations.

It was alleged that:

1. she failed to take a swab of a spot near to the intended incision line (for a hip replacement) or failed to ensure that a report was obtained from the pathology laboratory on the swab
2. she failed to inform a member of the medical staff that there was a spot
3. she failed to record her observation of the spot
4. she put a patient in jeopardy by giving false information to a surgeon about to operate, and
5. she forged a pathology report form

The nurse denied any responsibility for *1*, *2* and *3*, but admitted *4* and *5*.

The picture that emerged in evidence was that she was summoned to the theatre to speak to an angry consultant about a patient who was already anaesthetised and positioned on the table. The consultant asked if the spot had been noticed, if a swab had been taken, and if a report had been received. The sister panicked. She did not really know the patient as she had just come back from holiday. She felt that the registrar and house surgeon should have noticed. She trusted her staff. Faced with the consultant she said that a swab had been taken and the report was negative. With that information the consultant proceeded with the operation.

The sister, however, on return to her ward, found that no swab had been taken and therefore no report received. She panicked further, and altered a negative report received in respect of another patient and placed it in the first patient's notes when he returned from theatre.

The registrar and house surgeon (who had said nothing during the conversation in the theatre) doubted the story about the swab, and after the operation list had finished investigated and found the deception. The patient came to no harm, but the sister was dismissed from her employment.

The Disciplinary Committee felt that it was unreasonable to bring charges *1*, *2* and *3* against her and dismissed them, but considered *4* and *5* to be professional misconduct.

Would you have made that decision? If so which of the available three decisions would you then have made about this nurse? Her career to that moment had apparently been exemplary.

CASE A14. DISCIPLINARY COMMITTEE—CONVICTION

A report was received about a 32-year-old SRN, who had been convicted at Crown Court of 'having been knowingly concerned in the fraudulent evasion of the prohibition on importation of a controlled drug'. She had pleaded guilty, and was sentenced to 18 months' imprisonment, suspended for 2 years.

She had trained in Australia, and subsequently applied for registration in Great Britain. The details of her training and experience, and the professional references received, were entirely satisfactory, so she had been accepted without further requirement. For 2 years she had worked in the same hospital in Great Britain.

The circumstances in this case were very unusual. The nurse had met an American man some months before, and had become completely infatuated with him. At the Disciplinary Committee hearing she said quite voluntarily that she had been vaguely aware that he had something to do with drugs, but such was her infatuation that it did not really seem to matter. After some time the man said that he had to travel abroad on business, and urged her to arrange a period of unpaid leave, so that she could travel to meet him in India at the conclusion of his business trip, where they would have a holiday. She arranged the holiday, was provided by the man with a return air ticket to India, and travelled as planned. For 6 weeks they travelled around India; he was apparently charm itself, spent a great deal of money on her, and gave her a good time. Having prepared the ground well by his considerable expenditure of money, the man asked her to carry some drugs for him. He did not intend that the drugs remain in the U.K.; he provided her with a further air ticket onward from London to the U.S.A. She said that at first she expressed unwillingness, but on the basis of her infatuation she conceded. She seemed not to have known exactly what drug or how much was involved, but did say that she felt rather worried as she saw the case being packed, and even more when carrying it. When asked whether the knowledge that she was carrying a lot of drugs illegally worried her, she answered frankly that she would have felt worried by the fact that she was carrying drugs at all, and the quantity would not have affected her judgement.

Whether she was simply unfortunate or something was known about the movement of these drugs is not known, but she was stopped when changing planes. The investigating officer from the customs and excise department gave evidence to the Disciplinary Committee, and said that the nurse was found to be carrying 20,000 Mandrax tablets. He emphasised that a) she did not know how much or what drug she was carrying and b) from the moment she realised she had been tricked and used she cooperated with the police in the U.K. and the U.S.A. He also pointed out that the sentence of the court was lenient for an offence of this nature, the judge being convinced that her story was genuine and recognising that her cooperation with the police in two continents resulted in the man concerned being detained.

At the time of the hearing she was not employed in nursing, having left and obtained other employment until the Committee made their decision. The professional references received when she applied for registration were excellent; so also were those taken up in respect of her employment in Britain, and a senior nursing officer took the trouble to travel many miles at her own expense to tell the Committee how very competent this nurse was. On the other hand, in answering the Committee's questions, it appeared that the social ramifications of this action had not been recognised by the nurse.

If you had been a member of the Disciplinary Committee which of the available three decisions would you have made?

CASE A15. DISCIPLINARY COMMITTEE—ALLEGATION

An SRN of 27 years' experience, and two newly qualified SENs, appeared before the Disciplinary Committee, having been jointly involved in some incidents in which diamorphine had been incorrectly recorded and administered. All three admitted the allegations.

The chain of events started when nurse *A* (the SRN, sister of a ward for terminally ill patients) recieved a new stock of diamorphine ampoules 10mg, and incorrectly entered it in the drug book on the diamorphine 5 mg page. The records following this entry show that on two occasions a patient prescibed injections of 10 mg diamorphine received *two* 10 mg ampoules on each occasion, one being given by nurse *B*, and the other by nurse *C*, sister *A* having acted as witness on both occasions.

Nurse *B* stated that at the time of administration she had believed that only one 10 mg had been used, but in the face of the evidence she accepted that this could not have been the case. Her evidence also showed that the record in the drug book had been fully completed by herself and sister *A* *before* the drug had actually been administered.

Nurse *C* had been under the impression that Narphen and diamorphine were prescibed for the patient in alternating doses. This had been the case, but the prescition for Narphen had been cancelled. (This cancellation was not very clear.) During the afternoon, the patient became restless and sister *A* instructed nurse *C* to prepare injections of diamorphine and Narphen to be given together. The injections were prepared by sister *A* and nurse *C* and presumably the quantity of diamorphine was again inadvertently doubled. Again, the records were fully completed *before* actual administration. The patient, however, died in the meantime and so nurse C disposed of the drugs, watched by sister A.

Both nurses B and C knew they were wrong to sign the drug book before administering the drugs, but sister A agreed that they were acting under her instructions 'to save time'. It was clear that both young nurses were more than a little intimidated by this sister, whom they described as brisk and efficient, but not a person whose actions they could challenge. Nurse C clearly felt guilty and ashamed of the part she had played in the second incident, in that, firstly, she had not questioned sister A about combining the two injections of Narphen and diamorphine and that, secondly, she had not asked sister for the drug book so that she could indicate that the drugs had been wasted. She thought that perhaps sister A had received a telephoned instruction from the doctor concerning the injections and assumed that the records would be amended later, but had not dared to mention either point as sister was not the sort of person you could question.

Two days after these incidents, someone told sister A about her error in the diamorphine entry, whereupon she transferred and backdated the records to the correct page of the book, but in such a way as to indicate not receipt of the now reduced stock of ampoules but receipt of the full stock, making four false entries to account for the four ampoules already used and ordering nurse B to sign for the administration, she herself signing as witness. She then amended the patient's treatment card, to indicate more administration of diamorphine than the doctor had prescribed to match the entries she now made in the drug book. Nurse B did not know about this last point, but it was evident that she had not been happy in signing the additional entry sister A had made, and in fact asked sister whether errors ought not to be corrected by the pharmacist. Sister A had replied No and her manner had discouraged nurse B from pursuing the matter further.

Sister A appeared not to understand why she should be at a Disciplinary Committee at all. She clearly regarded the episode as an error in record-keeping which she had simply corrected. Although she admitted the allegations, she seemed not to believe it important that an incorrect quantity of diamorphine had been administered or that she was wrong to administer the diamorphine and Narphen together.

All three had been retained in employment. The SENs received counselling and were both adamant that in future when something appeared incorrect they would question it. The sister received 'counselling and retraining' before being re-allocated as a second sister on a training ward in a different hospital.

If you were a member of the Disciplinary Committee, what decision would you take in respect of each nurse?

CASE A16. DISCIPLINARY COMMITTEE—ALLEGATION

An SRN (aged 47) of many years experience appeared to answer a charge that she was guilty of misconduct, having failed to use her professional knowledge or exercise her professional judgement, as a result of which a patient she knew to be approximately 8 weeks' pregnant was given an injection of live attenuated rubella vaccine which had not been properly prescribed.

The SRN concerned (an employee of an AHA) had been employed as a district nurse attached to a group practice for $4\frac{1}{2}$ years at the time of the incident, having previously been employed as a district nurse/midwife in the same town for 2 years. Being attached to the practice, she undertook certain work on the surgery premises, and other in patients' homes. On occasions she was responsible for student nurses' community experience.

The incident had occurred 4 months earlier. A patient of the practice (a school teacher), believing that she was pregnant, rang the practice to tell them, and was told by the receptionist to bring in a urine specimen for testing. This she did, and was told to ring for the result. She rang and was told that her pregnancy was confirmed. The patient then told the receptionist that there was German measles in the school, and suggested she should have a test to assess her immunity. The receptionist told her to come at a certain time several days later.

In this practice it was the custom for the nurse to have a 'clinic' for 30–45 minutes each morning, which involved dressings, vaccine administration, and the like. The bookings were written by the receptionists in The Nurses' Book. The entry for this patient was written simply as: 'Mrs. XYZ—Rubella'.

The nurse observed (the day before the incident) this entry in her book, and in conversation with her midwife colleague learnt that the patient was in early pregnancy, and suggested that in that case she should be on the midwife's list. The next day, however, the name remained on her list, and the patient arrived. The patient proferred the inner aspect of her arm for blood to be taken, but the nurse turned the arm to administer an intramuscular injection, having taken the entry to mean that the patient had to have rubella vaccine. The patient drew her arm away (and the vaccine was wasted), saying as she did that she thought she had to have blood taken. The nurse called the reception desk where it was busy and noisy, and believed that she was first told they would check with a doctor, and then that the receptionist indicated the doctor had said the patient was to have the injection. The nurse then took another phial of vaccine, told the patient that it had been checked with the doctor, and administered it.

In evidence before the Committee it was learnt that the patient had not seen a doctor, and that there had been no check with a doctor on the day. The receptionist indicated that normally she would have written 'Blood for rubella antibodies' in the book in these circumstances. Two days later one of the doctors contacted the patient to say that there had been a ghastly mistake. The 35-year-old woman decided that her much wanted first pregnancy should be terminated.

The Committee noted the absence of good practices and policies in this surgery, and the inadequacy of contact with and oversight from the nursing officer and senior nursing officer. The nurse had two toenails removed during her preceding days off, and had returned to duty (in some pain) against her husband's wishes because staff would have been short. Her record in this area had been good, and since the incident she had been moved to a post as second sister in a geriatric ward.

The complaint alleging professional misconduct had been brought to the Council by the patient's husband. The nurse admitted the facts of the charge and clearly was extremely sorry.

You are the Disciplinary Committee. Would you have regarded this as professional misconduct? If Yes, which of the three available decisions would you then have made?

CASE A17. DISCIPLINARY COMMITTEE—ALLEGATION

A report was received about an incident in a general hospital which had resulted in the death of a 13-year-old girl less than 9 hours after an operation to remove her appendix. This became an allegation case before the Disciplinary Committee. Those against whom allegations were brought to the Committee were (i) the night nursing officer (hereafter called nurse *A*); (ii) a staff nurse (nurse *B*); (iii) a state enrolled nurse (nurse *C*);and (iv) a state enrolled nurse doing student nurse training (nurse *D*).

The picture that emerged in evidence was:

The 13-year-old girl, was admitted with appendicitis, and was in the operating theatre at the time the night staff came on duty. A little while later they collected her from theatre, and subsequently gave her an intramuscular injection of pethidine 50 mg. She settled down well, but in the early hours of the morning she woke, and was troubled by persistent vomiting.

Nurse *C* telephoned nurse *A*, who told her to come to her with the patient's prescription card. This she did, and nurse *A* noted that the child was written up for one further injection of pethidine. She considered this inappropriate for the symptoms described, so she telephoned the house surgeon. (The time was now 4:00 A.M.) He told her that the child should be given an intramuscular injection of Maxolon 10 mg. Nurse *A* passed this instruction to nurse *C*, but she did not write it down. She added that nurse *C* would not have it on her ward, so she should go to another specific ward to get some.

Nurse *C* went to the other ward as instructed (but with no written instruction), where she met nurse *B*. Nurse *B* was in conversation in the office with a colleague. Nurse *C* put her verbal request to nurse *B*, who went to the drug cupboard in a dim corner of the office. She opened the cupboard, and saw that there was a box of Maxolon ampoules, and some loose ampoules beside it. Nurse *B* took two of the loose ampoules (having assumed them to be Maxolon) and, without really interrupting her conversation, gave them to nurse *C*, who received them in the belief that they were the drug that she had been instructed to obtain and give.

Nurse *C* returned to her own ward, where she explained to her colleague nurse *D* what had transpired. Meanwhile the patient was still vomiting. Together nurses *C* and *D* drew up the contents of the two ampoules they had been given. They remarked that the quantity of the two ampoules together came to 8 mg, when nurse *A* had said 10 mg. They also expressed surprise that it amounted to a 4-ml injection, which they considered a lot for the patient. Finally, they noticed that the name on the ampoules was Pavulon, and not that stated by nurse *A*, but they knew from their previous experience that there was often more than one brand name for the same drug. Together they made their way towards the patient's bed.

It was a busy night on this large surgical ward, and the staff of two had a lot to cope with. At this stage another patient rang and called for urgent attention, so nurse *D* went to answer the call. Nurse *C* continued and gave the injection of Pavulon. She recorded the fact that the drug had been given. Nurse *D* signed as having witnessed it, although she had not done so. They noted that their patient settled down well. AT 6:00 A.M. they found her dead. The subsequent investigations revealed that the drug given was not Maxolon.

The official document in use in the particular health authority concerning the control and administration of drugs required that the administration be witnessed by a second person, and that both signatures be recorded. The document made no reference to a prodecure to be followed where a drug was verbally ordered at night.

In this case the allegations were all admitted. The Disciplinary Committee had to decide whether each nurse was guilty of misconduct, and if Yes, what to do about it. What would your decision have been?

CASE A18. DISCIPLINARY COMMITTEE—CONVICTION

An RMN, aged 28 years, was brought to the attention of the Council by the police, having been convicted of unlawful sexual intercourse with a patient, contrary to Section 128 of the Mental Health Act. He had been placed on probation for 2 years, and his employment had been terminated.

Evidence presented at the hearing made it clear that the patient had been admitted because her behaviour became intolerable to her family. She boasted of her sexual promiscuity. She had come to the hospital from a remand centre, and was admitted to the Therapeutic Community Unit to see if this would achieve the breakthrough which more authoritarian settings had failed to achieve.

The consultant psychiatrist explained in writing that the unit was the complete reverse of authoritarian, that nurses were discouraged from wearing their uniforms, and encouraged to form personal relationships with patients. ('To see them all the time as persons *and* patients' was how he summed it up.)

Meanwhile the RMN's marriage was in some difficulty, and a relationship began. No one in authority became aware of the situation until it was too late. No sexual intercourse took place in hospital premises. The degree to which the relationship had developed became clear (and resulted in the charge and conviction) when the nurse's wife came home to their flat unexpectedly and found a naked woman in the spare room. The wife reported the situation to the nursing administrators at the hospital, who in their turn called the police.

The case was forwarded to the Disciplinary Committee for a hearing. The nurse attended the meeting with his probation officer, and impressed the Committee by his attitude. Letters were received from several psychiatrists and senior nursing staff, all were complimentary about his competence as a psychiatric nurse, and expressed their regret that his vulnerability in these particular circumstances had not been noticed. They now felt that he needed a more authoritarian setting to work to his fullest capacity.

If you had been a member of the Disciplinary Committee what decision would you have made?

CASE A19. DISCIPLINARY COMMITTEE—APPLICATION FOR ENROLMENT

In the period between submitting an entry for the pupil nurse assessment and receiving the letter to indicate that he had been successful, a pupil nurse who had been training for the part of the Roll for Nurses of the Mentally Subnormal was convicted in court of the theft of a small sum of money from a fund held at ward level for patients' sweets and tobacco. In consequence of his conviction his employment had been terminated.

Since the young man concerned had completed the statutory training period and passed the required practical tests, he was eligible to apply for enrolment when he received a letter to indicate that he had passed the assessment. The director of nurse education confirmed the completion date and that, until this incident, the conduct and competence of this pupil nurse had been very good. He was described as being very pleasant and caring.

In his letter to the Investigating Committee the pupil nurse expressed his remorse and shame about this lapse that occurred in a moment of weakness when his personal finances were in something of a mess. The Investigating Committee (who can either accept an application for enrolment or refer it to the Disciplinary Committee) felt unable to accept the application since the part of the Roll concerned gave this man access only to a particularly vulnerable group of patients.

The matter was therefore referred to the Disciplinary Committee for a hearing. At that time the young man had obtained employment in an ironmongers' shop, having told the owner of his problem. He was also working voluntarily in his spare time in a club for the mentally handicapped, and here also the officers knew about his conviction and had written to the Committee with a very favourable report on his work for their caring organisation.

The Disciplinary Committee were impressed by the remorse shown by the man, and by his determination to repay the debt he felt he owed to society and the mentally handicapped.

The Committee are able to say Yes or No to the application, but if they say No it is normal for them to indicate when they would reconsider the application and to set any special conditions.

As a member of the Disciplinary Committee what decision would you recommend to your colleagues?

CASE A20. INVESTIGATING COMMITTEE—SRN/STUDENT NURSE IN TRAINING

A student nurse in training for the part of the Register for Mental Nurses, who was also an SRN of about 2 years' standing, was the subject of consideration by the Investigating Committee. She admitted to them in writing that she had been found collapsed and ill in a corridor of the nurses residence, that by the time help was summoned she was deeply unconscious, and that these circumstances resulted from her ingesting a large amount of hypnotic drugs that she had misappropriated from the ward to which she was allocated.

The Investigating Committee members had to make decisions on her status as a registered nurse and her position as a potential examination entrant. On the first point they could (a) decide that the matter was of no concern to the nursing profession (b) caution and counsel by letter, or (c) refer the case to the Disciplinary Committee. On the second point they could close the matter immediately or ask that it come back to them when an examination application was actually received.

There were a number of tragic factors in the personal life of this nurse that led her to take the action she admitted. One was that her fiancé had recently been killed in a road accident. Another was the prolonged suffering of her father who was in a terminal illness of malignant cause. All the evidence showed that until these problems affected her life she had been an excellent staff nurse and student nurse.

In the short term the nurse was provided with the necessary resuscitative treatment and longer term medical and psychiatric help while on sick leave. The director of nurse education reported the matter quickly to the Council because he considered it his professional responsibility to do so, and because he realised that this would also open the way to an offer of additional support from a professional social worker on the staff of the Nurses Welfare Service.

It was therefore some months later that the case actually came before the Investigating Committee for which occasion there were available not only helpful medical and psychiatric reports but a social enquiry report from the Welfare Service.

You are the Investigating Committee. In respect of the SRN status you can say:

a. it is of no concern *or*

b. you can caution and counsel *or*

c. you can send it to the Disciplinary Committee.

In respect of her position as a student nurse:

a. you can close the matter *or*

b. you can ask to consider it again when she submits an examination entry *or*

c. you can terminate her training.

What will you do?

CASE A21. DISCIPLINARY COMMITTEE—CONVICTION

A SRN, aged 38 years, was reported to the Council having been found guilty of obtaining a quantity of Nembutal tablets valued at 20 pence by virtue of a forged prescription with intent to defraud.

She was a district nurse attached to a busy group general practice. She had a deep vein thrombosis and was advised by her doctor (from another practice) to stop working for 7 days. In association with this condition she had difficulty in sleeping and was prescribed Nembutal.

She again suffered with deep vein thrombosis but continued working as the practice was so busy and the pressure of work great. She had a husband and 4 children of school age, and was studying to take further examinations. As a result of these pressures, she said she did not have time to visit her doctor (who was several miles away) for renewal of her prescription, and so added Nembutal to a prescription prepared for a patient which was then signed by the doctor for whom she worked.

The fact that one item in the prescription was in a different writing was noticed by the dispensing chemist who informed the doctor, to whom the nurse admitted what she had done and explained the circumstances. He felt it his duty to inform her own GP who said the only crime she was guilty of was that of putting her patients before herself. Having at first said it would go no further the GP felt he ought to report it to the district community physician. In consequence she was dismissed from her employment as well as found guilty in court. However, on appeal to the Area Health Authority she was reinstated.

She had been nursing for 20 years, and the documents assembled from senior nursing personnel on her career showed it to have been exemplary.

She had had a very bad spell all within a period of 1 year, with the work load, family commitments, studying and also the death of her youngest brother, aged 25 years. Three days after his death, his widow committed suicide, leaving a 6-month-old baby. Her decision not to adopt the child was a hard one to make and left her feeling that she had let her brother down.

She impressed the Committee as an extremely competent and caring registered nurse, who fully realised the significance of the action which lead to her appearance in court. She had realised that she was over-committed, and had discontinued the studies which had been part of the exceptionally heavy load. Her reinstatement had been to the same group practice.

If you had been a member of the Disciplinary Committee what decision would you have made?

CASE A22. INVESTIGATING COMMITTEE—ALLEGATION

A 40-year-old Registered Nurse for the Mentally Subnormal was the subject of allegations to the General Nursing Council for England and Wales (as were other nurses from the hospital where he was a charge nurse on night duty) to the effect that he had absented himself from duty without good reason, as a result of which mentally subnormal patients were put at risk.

The circumstances were that, because of incidents during the day, there had been a union meeting which led to a call for industrial action. The nurse knew nothing of this until he came to the hospital to begin his night-duty shift. He was met by officials concerned with the strike which had commenced in the afternoon. Having heard their explanation he went to the wards he would be covering to ascertain for himself the adequacy of the cover, and talked to a nursing officer on the matter.

He found that the patients were well settled for the night and that the coverage (in the form of a nursing officer who had stayed on duty, and a number of volunteers) was adequate for the quiet hours of the night, and so went to the building where those who had withdrawn their labour had gathered.

As the night progressed he reasoned with himself that while the staff and volunteers could manage for the quiet hours, it would be impossible for them to cope when morning came and the mentally handicapped residents had to be identified for medications, diets, and the like. He therefore returned to take up his duties well before those residents would be waking, and continued to the end of his shift. The strike was called off by the next night.

When dealing with an allegation case the Investigating Committee must decide that:

a. the nurse had no case to answer *or*

b. the admitted allegations constitute misconduct, but that a letter of admonition and counsel will suffice *or*

c. the allegations, if proved, constitute professional misconduct in their opinion, and justify a hearing before the Disciplinary Committee.

Which would you choose in this case?

Appendix B

Decisions and Comments for Case Studies

For each case in Appendix A and those contained within the various chapters of the book (where the Committee's decision was not made known) I set out the decision made by the Committee which dealt with the case, and add some explanatory comments. Again, for easy reference, there is a Table of Cases on page 155.

If you disagree with the decision remember that the Committee members who dealt with the case had more information than was given to you, and that, if it was a Disciplinary Committee case, they had probably met the nurse concerned.

Bear in mind also that the Committees are composed of people like you, from different backgrounds of training, experience and bias, and that the decisions were made by simple majority votes with no abstentions allowed.

CASE A1

Case A1 is an example at one and the same time of two areas of concern to the General Nursing Council for England and Wales which have been expressed through its annual reports of 1977–78 and 1978–79.

The nurse received a *postponed judgement* decision for a 1-year period. During that year she had further surgery which at last resolved her health problem. When she attended the resumed hearing of the case she was a more healthy and confident person, no longer requiring any analgesic drugs. She had been employed in nursing again for 3 months, and the evidence was that she was enjoying it and performing to the entire satisfaction of her managers.

The Committee therefore resolved to administer a caution and close the case.

CASE A2

Case A2 is an example of the considerable number that are seen wherein a nurse has committed some professionally reprehensible actions against a background of domestic disharmony. In this type of case attendance at the hearing is of the greatest importance. In this case it certainly prevented the

137

Committee from deciding to remove the man's name from the Register.
The Committee administered a *very stern caution*.

CASE A3

The committees have to deal with large numbers of cases involving theft from
hospitals and a smaller (though still significant) number involving theft from
patients. This case was a little of the former with more of the latter, and also a
theft from a colleague. On the face of it the picture for her looked very bleak.

The fact, however, that it was all out of character, that she recognised fully
the significance of her reprehensible actions, that she was again on an even
keel, and that she had worked hard to repay her debt to society were all
important.

It was a case in which the respondent nurse's attendance was crucial,
because the judgement of individual members on her as a person was influenced by her answers to their searching questions.

The Committee decided to administer a *very stern caution*.

CASE A4

I hope that you have noted and considered some of the underlying reasons for
the appalling fracas contained in case A4.

The SEN was *removed from the Roll* of Nurses. The SRN was made the
subject of a *postponed judgement* decision for 1 year.

CASE A5

A considerable number of cases prove to be either the result of or set against
the background of serious disharmony in a close personal relationship. Case
A5 is one such example, and as is often the case the person involved was clearly
a nurse of high standards and considerable commitment. (It is the very level of
the commitment to professional work that often triggers the disharmony, as it
did here.)

Much affected by the various reports, the Committee decided to *postpone
judgement* for 1 year. She obtained nursing employment elsewhere in the same
area very quickly. There was another crisis in her marriage leading to its
breakdown, but she managed to survive without further 'professional' offence
and see the postponed judgement period conclude safely.

CASE A6

The importance of attendance at the Committee has been emphasised; it can
rarely have been as important as in case A6.

The nurse impressed the Committee members as enormously as she had the
divisional nursing officer. They decided to administer a *very stern caution*.

CASE A7

The Investigating Committee opted for decision *b*.

CASE A8

Note how marital disharmony, this time fired by alcohol abuse, lay behind this nurse's actions—actions which she clearly regretted for all the right reasons.

The Committee administered a *very stern caution*.

CASE A9

The Council have twice mentioned in their annual reports to the secretary of state that the incidence of unfitness on duty due to alcohol is disturbingly high. It usually involves female nurses.

In this case, noting (a) that the nurse was now receiving specialist treatment and (b) that she did not intend to seek nursing employment until the specialist felt it safe to do so, the Committee decided to *postpone judgement* for 1 year, and to require reports from the psychiatrist and her general practitioner for the resumed hearing.

CASE A10

In Chapter 9 I have referred to cases that arise out of the extension of the nurse's role—this is an example.

The Committee could not seem really to get to understand this nurse's actions, as she seemed to keep them at a distance throughout the hearing.

The Committee decided to *remove her name from the Register of Nurses*. Rather than seem angry, bitter or frustrated at that decision, she actually seemed relieved.

CASE A11

In Case A11 the man had been convicted of a gravely serious act of 'wounding with intent'. His only qualification enabled him to work in potentially provocative situations. The incident had happened only 7 months after he became an enrolled nurse. The Valium possession seemed to indicate a lack of responsibility.

The Committee decided to *remove his name from the Roll of Nurses*.

CASE A12

Case A12 provides an example of the quite significant number of cases from mental subnormality hospitals. In this one, as so often, the staffing level was disturbingly low. The patients/residents, however, are extremely vulnerable, and the evidence of the fabricated story was disturbing.

The decision was made to *remove her name from the Register*.

CASE A13

Case A13 seems to say a great deal about relationships in the hospital where it occurred.

The Committee were impressed by this nurse, though deploring her foolish and reckless action. She was given a *postponed judgement* decision for 1 year. She quickly found new nursing employment with managers in whom she confided. The period of postponed judgement was very satisfactorily concluded.

CASE A14

Case A14 presented the Committee with something of an enigma—an apparently good nurse, but one gullible enough to be lured into trafficking in drugs on this scale.

Not without some feelings of regret, the Committee decided to *remove her name from the Register of Nurses*. She has subsequently been restored, clearly a more wise and mature person.

CASE A15

Case A15 is really three cases in one, and, I suggest, a case worth much study and discussion. The events occurred in a remote hospital with no on-site pharmacy. The sister had been in the employment of this authority and trusted for many years, and they had not dismissed her. (Was this perhaps a recognition of their guilt for not exercising proper oversight?)

In the event the Committee felt that the newly qualified *enrolled nurses* were victims of the situation in which they found themselves, and had learnt from the experience. They each received a *caution only*. The SRN provided more of a problem to the Committee. Eventually, noting that her employers had engaged in 'retraining' they decided to *postpone judgement* for 1 year, with the rider that the authority look again at the adequacy of that retraining/counselling.

CASE A16

Case A16 is a case of importance for many reasons. It was a 'private citizen' complaint. The nurse was working in a bad setting that was not really of her making, and received little or no support from her managers. In that setting sound policies seemed nonexistent. Nonetheless the nurse had failed to use her professional knowledge or exercise her professional judgement, and a tragedy resulted.

Had it not been for the mitigation to be found in the inadequacies of others I would imagine that 'removal' might have been the decision. As it was the Committee *postponed judgement* for 1 year.

CASE A17

Case A17 is four cases in one in a tragic chain of events. The absence of any clear policy and procedure in respect of verbal ordering of drugs was a crucial feature of this case, and assisted the nursing officer's representative. Against that, she had sent an enrolled nurse on her way to obtain a drug with nothing to check it against—very disturbing!

This case came before a new Committee on their first day, and left them wondering just what they had committed themselves to.

Postponed judgement decisions were made for nurses *A*, *B* and *C*. Nurse *D* was the subject of a *caution*.

CASE A18

Cases like A18 often stem from therapeutic community units. In this case we see the matching of the nurse who needed a more authoritarian setting with the patient who also needed a more authoritarian setting.

The decision was to *postpone judgement* for the duration of the probation order. Both the probation order and postponed judgement period came to a satisfactory close about 9 months later.

CASE A19

Case A19 is an example of how the route to the Register or Roll is controlled. This case required you to answer the question 'Would you admit this person to the Roll of Nurses?

The Committee's decision was that they would not at that stage, but would be willing to reconsider if he applied in not less than 6 months and could provide references from people with knowledge of the facts. He applied again about 9 months later, was again well supported, and was accepted.

CASE A20

Basically A20 is a case of sickness rather than badness, and an example of good managerial support.

In respect of her SRN status option *b* was chosen. In respect of her student nurse status the second option *b* was chosen. She resumed her training and was successful, and the director of nurse education was fully vindicated.

CASE A21

The nurse in Case A21 committed a foolish offence at a difficult time in her life. The Committee chose to *administer a caution*.

CASE A22

In Case A22 the Committee decided that the nurse had no case to answer. Some others involved in the same incident but who had acted with less responsibility were forwarded to the Disciplinary Committee for hearings.

CASE 5 (CHAPTER 2)

The nurse entered the committee room in a confident manner, his representative having told him what he then put to the Committee: that it was a minor drug and that it only warranted a caution. The Committee, however, were concerned about the attitudes it betrayed and the method of obtaining the drug. The nurse, his confidence and complacency much disturbed by the penetrating questions of the Committee, just about avoided removal, and was placed on *postponed judgement*. With a great deal of help from the Welfare Service he was able to use this period to gain in maturity, insight and knowledge.

CASE 6 (CHAPTER 2)

Case 6 was placed before the Investigating Committee only when various medical and social work reports were available. The Committee saw the nurse as a victim, and were pleased with the evidence that she was well again. They required a letter conveying a *mild caution*.

CASE 8 (CHAPTER 2)

The nurse who was the subject of Case 8 was *removed from the Register*.

CASE 9 (CHAPTER 5)

Case 9 provides another example of the machinery that allows control of the route to the Register or Roll of Nurses. Into the scales went this proven reprehensible action against the support of the director of nurse education and a number of excellent ward reports. The Committee decided to allow the examination entry, but gave the pupil nurse a *very stern caution*.

CASE 11 (CHAPTER 6)

The text explains the Case 11. The nurse was placed on *postponed judgement*, and the period was successfully concluded.

Appendix C

Professional Discipline Statistics 1978–79

The professional discipline statistics for the year 1978–79 relate only to the General Nursing Council for England and Wales. The tables show total figures of cases, decisions and offences for the Investigating Committee (A1–A4) and for the Disciplinary Committee (A5–A9). The number of offences is sometimes more than the number of cases because the nurse who is the subject of a case may have committed more than one offence.

1. INVESTIGATING COMMITTEE

TABLE A1. Cases and decisions: qualified nurses.

Nurse status	Conviction decisions						Allegation decisions						Total
	No action		Depre-cated		Referred to DC		No case		Depre-cated		Referred to DC		
	F	M	F	M	F	M	F	M	F	M	F	M	
Registered	21	19	46	29	41	19	25	8	6	2	23	10	249
Enrolled	13	3	55	16	12	12	9	3	4		15	3	145
Registered & Enrolled		1	2	2	1		2		1		1	2	12
Total	34	23	103	47	54	31	36	11	11	2	39	15	406

DC = Disciplinary Committee

TABLE A2. Cases and decisions: learner nurses.

Learner status	Conviction cases								Allegation cases								Total	
	No action		AA		Application referred to DC		Training extended		No case		AA		Application referred to DC		Training extended			
	F	M	F	M	F	M	F	M	F	M	F	M	F	M	F	M	F	M
Student	21	6	11	13	1	2			2								56	
Pupil	4	3	3	1	2		2	2				1		1	1	1	21	
Total	25	9	14	14	3	2	2	2	2			1		1	1	1	77	

AA = applications accepted
DC = Disciplinary Committee

TABLE A3. Offences and decisions: qualified nurses.

Offences	Total Offences		Conviction decisions						Allegation decisions					
			No action		Deprecated		Forwarded to DC		No case		Deprecated		Forwarded to DC	
	F	M	F	M	F	M	F	M	F	M	F	M	F	M
DRUG OFFENCES														
Cannabis	6	6			3	3	3	3	1				1	
Forgery	10	1			1		5	6			2	1	9	3
Theft	25	10					15			1	1		1	
Theft and false entry	3						1		1		2		2	
Other	12	4			2	1	3	3	3					
Total	56	21			6	4	27	12	5	1	5	1	13	3
NURSING OFFENCES														
Falsely claiming other nursing qualifications	2						2							
Nursing practice	32	9							21	3	2	1	9	5
Unfit for duty due to drinks/drugs	12	6							2	4			10	
Other professional misconduct	12								9				3	2
Total	58	15					2		32	7	2	1	22	7

TABLE A 3 *continued.*   Offences and decisions: qualified nurses.

Offence	Total											
PATIENT ABUSE												
Drug	1	1									1	1
Physical	6	12									4	6
Sexual	2	5									2	3
Theft from patients	9	4										
Total	18	22									7	10
THEFT AND OTHER DISHONESTY												
Hospital property	16	6										
Obtaining by deception	17	7										
Shoplifting	75	10										
Other theft	11	5										
Total	119	28										
MISCELLANEOUS OFFENCES												
Alcohol offences	4	4										
Assault	7	7										
Fraudulent travel	9	4										
Motor vehicle offences	13	4										
Sexual offences	1	13										
Other offences	96	18										
Total	130	50										
GRAND TOTAL	381	136	35	19	108	46	48	13	11	3	47	22

DC = Disciplinary Committee

TABLE A4. Offences and decisions: learner nurses.

Cases	Total offences		Conviction decisions								Allegation decisions							
			No action		AA		Referred to DC		Training extended		No case		AA		Referred to DC		Training extended	
	F	M	F	M	F	M	F	M	F	M	F	M	F	M	F	M	F	M
DRUG OFFENCES																		
Cannabis	2	3			1	2		1		1								
Forgery	1				1													
Theft	2				1							1						
Other	1	1				1				1								
Total	6	4			3	3		1		2		1						
NURSING OFFENCES																		
Falsely claiming other nursing qualifications		1														1		
Nursing practice		1														1		
Total		2														2		

TABLE A4 *continued.* Offences and decisions: learner nurses.

PATIENT ABUSE												
Sexual	1											1
Total	1											1
THEFT AND OTHER DISHONESTY												
Hospital property	1		1									
Obtaining by deception	3	2	1		1	2	1	1				
Shoplifting	10	2			7	2	2	1				
Other theft	2	7			2	4	2			2		
Total	16	11	1		11	6	3	2		2	2	1
MISCELLANEOUS OFFENCES												
Assault	1	2			1	2	1	2				
Fraudulent travel	16	2	14	2	2	2						
Motor vehicle offences	6	4	6		1		1		1			
Sexual offences	1				1			1				1
Other offences	7	9	4	5	1	2	1	2	1	1	1	1
Total	30	18	24	9	4	6	2	5	2	2	1	1
GRAND TOTAL	52	36	25	9	18	15	3	5	2	2	2	4	1

AA = application accepted
DC = Disciplinary Committee

2. DISCIPLINARY COMMITTEE

TABLE A5. Total new cases and decisions: qualified nurses.

Nurse status	Conviction cases						Allegation cases								Total
	Caution		Postpone judgement		Remove		Not proved		Caution		Postpone judgement		Remove		
	F	M	F	M	F	M	F	M	F	M	F	M	F	M	
Registered	12	2	12	5	13	6	3	1	7	2	6	3	4	4	80
Enrolled	4	1	1	5	7	9	2		2		3	2	6	3	45
Registered & Enrolled											1				1
Total	16	3	13	10	20	15	5	1	9	2	10	5	10	7	126

TABLE A6. Total resumed cases and decisions: qualified nurses.

Nurse status	Postponed judgement						Applications for restoration				Total
	Caution		Further postpone judgement		Remove		Application accepted		Application refused		
	F	M	F	M	F	M	F	M	F	M	
Registered	10	8				1	10	3	1		33
Enrolled	2	2	2	1	2	1	1		2		13
Registered & Enrolled	1	4									5
Total	13	14	2	1	2	2	13	3	3		51

TABLE A7. Total cases and decisions: learner nurses.

Learner status	Conviction cases				Allegation cases				Total
	Application accepted		Application refused		Application accepted		Application refused		
	F	M	F	M	F	M	F	M	
Student	1	1		2					4
Pupil	2					1			3
Total	3	1		2		1			7

TABLE A8. Offences and decisions (new and resumed cases): qualified nurses.

			New cases												Resumed cases						
	Total offences		Conviction decisions			Allegation decisions						Postponed judgements			Applications for restoration			
			Caution	Postponed judgement	Remove	Not proved	Caution	Postponed judgement	Remove	Total new cases		Caution	Further postponed judgement	Remove	Accepted	Refused	Total resumed cases
	F M	F M	F M	F M	F M	F M	F M	F M	F M	F M	F M	F M	F M	F M	F M	F M
DRUG OFFENCES																
Cannabis	3 5	4	2 2	2					2 4	1			1		1 1
Forgery	9		1	2					8	1			1		1 1
Theft	42 12	6	5	6		5 1	6	3 1	31 8	5 4		1	4	1	11 4
Theft and false entry	4			1					2				1		2
Other	5 7	1	1 1	2 2				1	4 3	1 4			1	1	1 4
Total	63 24	11	9 3	11 10		5 1	7	4 1	47 15	8 8		1	6 1	1	16 9
NURSING OFFENCES																
Falsely claiming other nursing qualifications	5	1			2 1	3 1		4 2	2	1	1		1		3
Nursing practice	10 6			1		1	1	4 2	9 5	1	1		1		1 1
Unfit for duty due to drink/drugs	13				1		3	5	10	1	1		1		3
Other professional misconduct	5 2				1	1		2 1	3 2	1			1		2
Total	33 8	1		1	4 1	4 2	3 1	11 3	24 7	3 1	2		4		9

TABLE A 8 *continued*. Offences and decisions: (new and resumed cases): qualified nurses.

Offence	Total												
PATIENT ABUSE													
Drugs	7 / 13	1				1 4	3 3 1		6 12 1			1	1 1
Physical	2 / 3		3	2 1			3 3	2 3	2 3				
Sexual				1 2									
Theft from patients	14 / 5	2 3	3 1	2 1	3	1 5	3 5	7 2	4 3	1	1 1	7 3
Total	23 / 22	3 3	3 4	2 4	3	1 5	5 18	5 3	1	1 1	8 4
THEFT AND OTHER DISHONESTY													
Hospital property	14 / 5	5 1	1 1	4 1			10 2	2 3	1	1	4 3
Obtaining by deception	14 / 4	2 1	3 1	5		1	11 1	1 3	1	1	3 3
Shoplifting	1						1				
Other theft	5 / 4	1	1	2 1			3 1	2	1	1	2 3
Total	34 / 13	8 1	5 1	11 2	1		25 4	3 8	1	3 2	9 9
MISCELLANEOUS OFFENCES													
Alcohol offences	1										
Assault	1 / 5	1	1	1			1 2	1	2	1	1 3
Fraudulent travel											
Motor vehicle offences	1 / 1		1	1						1	1
Sexual offences	5	1 1		2	1		2	1		1	1 3
Other offences	7 / 6	1	1	3 2			6 5	1	1	1	1 1
Total	10 / 16	1 2	2 1	3 4	1		2 7 9	3	1	1 3 2	3 7
GRAND TOTAL	163 / 83	24 3	19 9	28 20	8 1	9 3	12 6	18 11	118 53	19 23	4 1	15 4 6	45 30

TABLE A9. Offences and decisions: learner nurses.

Cases	Total offences		Conviction decisions				Allegation decisions			
			Application accepted		Application refused		Application accepted		Application refused	
	F	M	F	M	F	M	F	M	F	M
DRUG OFFENCES										
Cannibis		1		1						
Total		1		1						
NURSING OFFENCES										
Falsely claiming other nursing qualifications		1						1		
Total		1						1		
PATIENT ABUSE										
Total										
THEFT AND OTHER DISHONESTY										
Obtaining by deception	1	3	1			2	1			
Shoplifting	2		2							
Other theft		2				2				
Total	3	5	3			4	1			
MISCELLANEOUS OFFENCES										
Motor vehicle offences		1	1							
Other offences		1				1				
Total		2	1			1				
GRAND TOTAL	3	9	3	2		5	2			

Table of Cases

Index

157